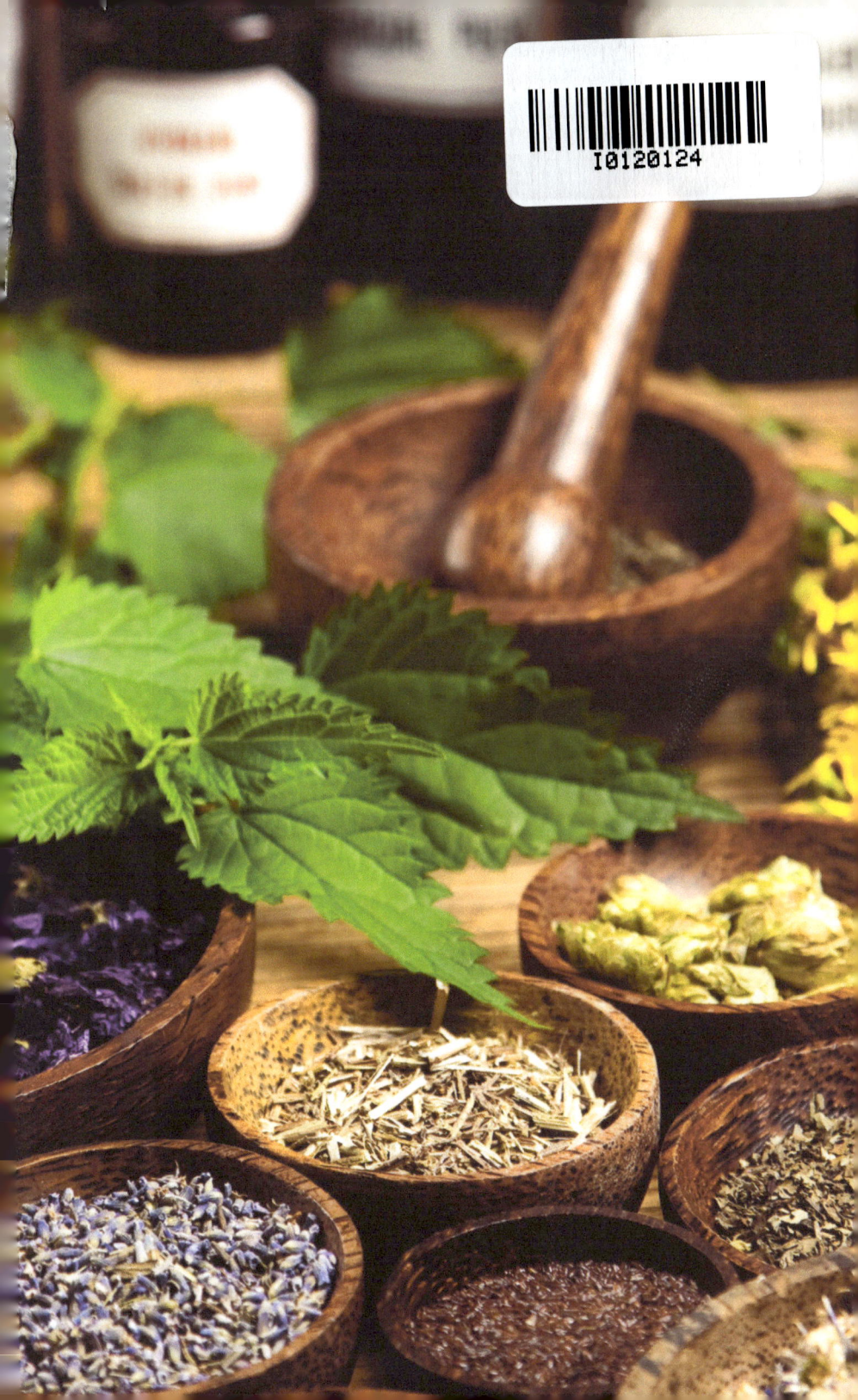

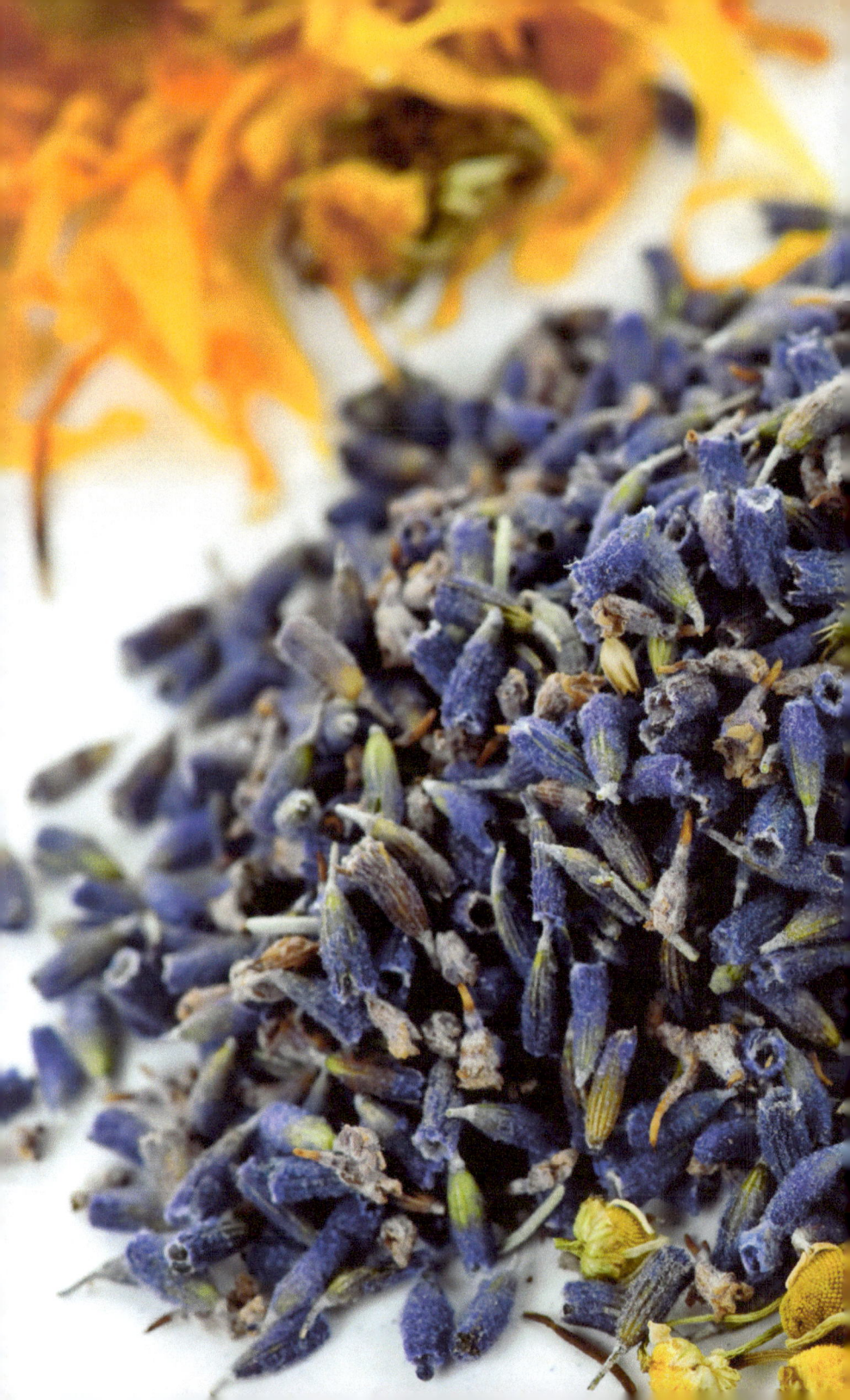

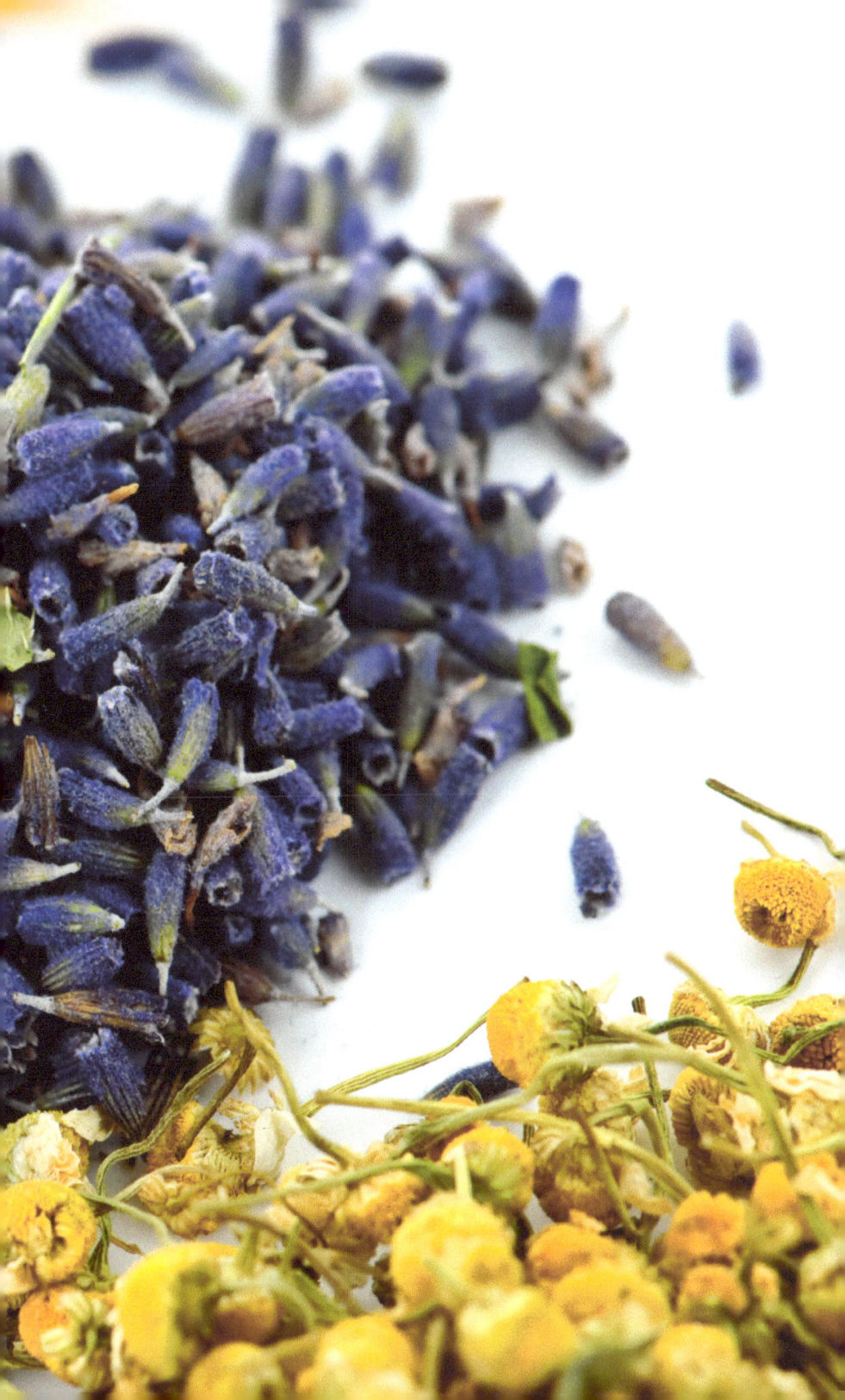

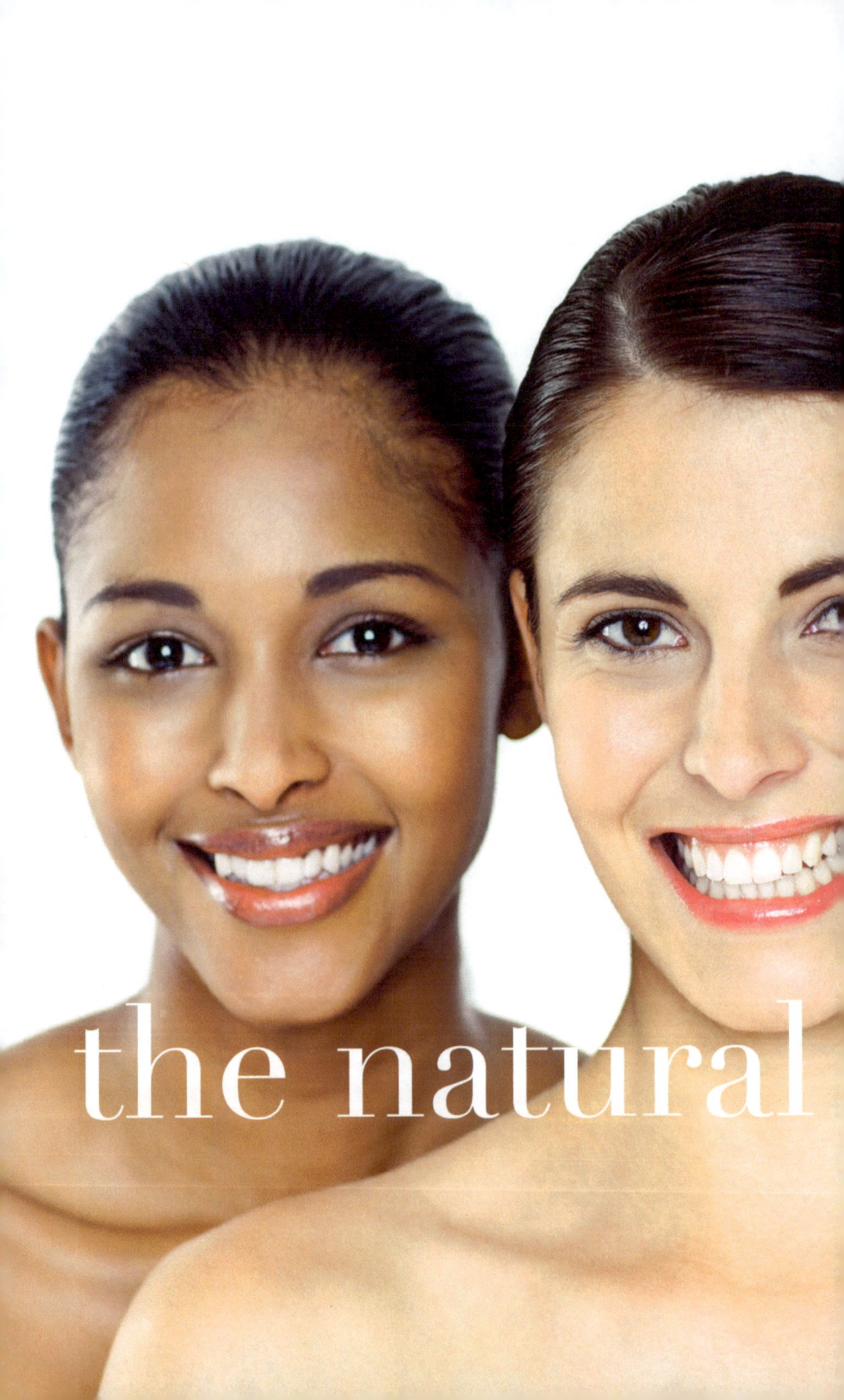

the natural

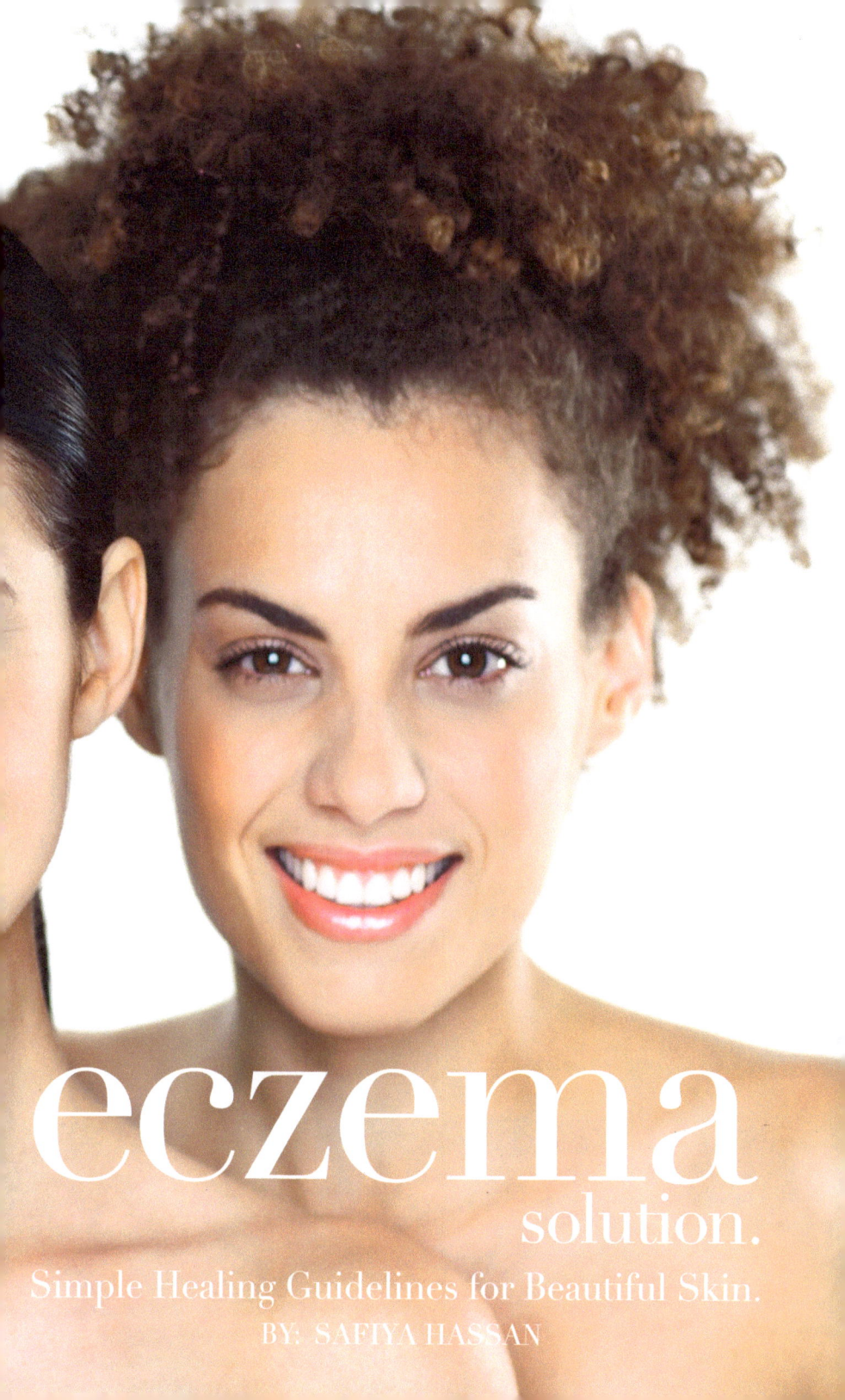

eczema
solution.

Simple Healing Guidelines for Beautiful Skin.
BY: SAFIYA HASSAN

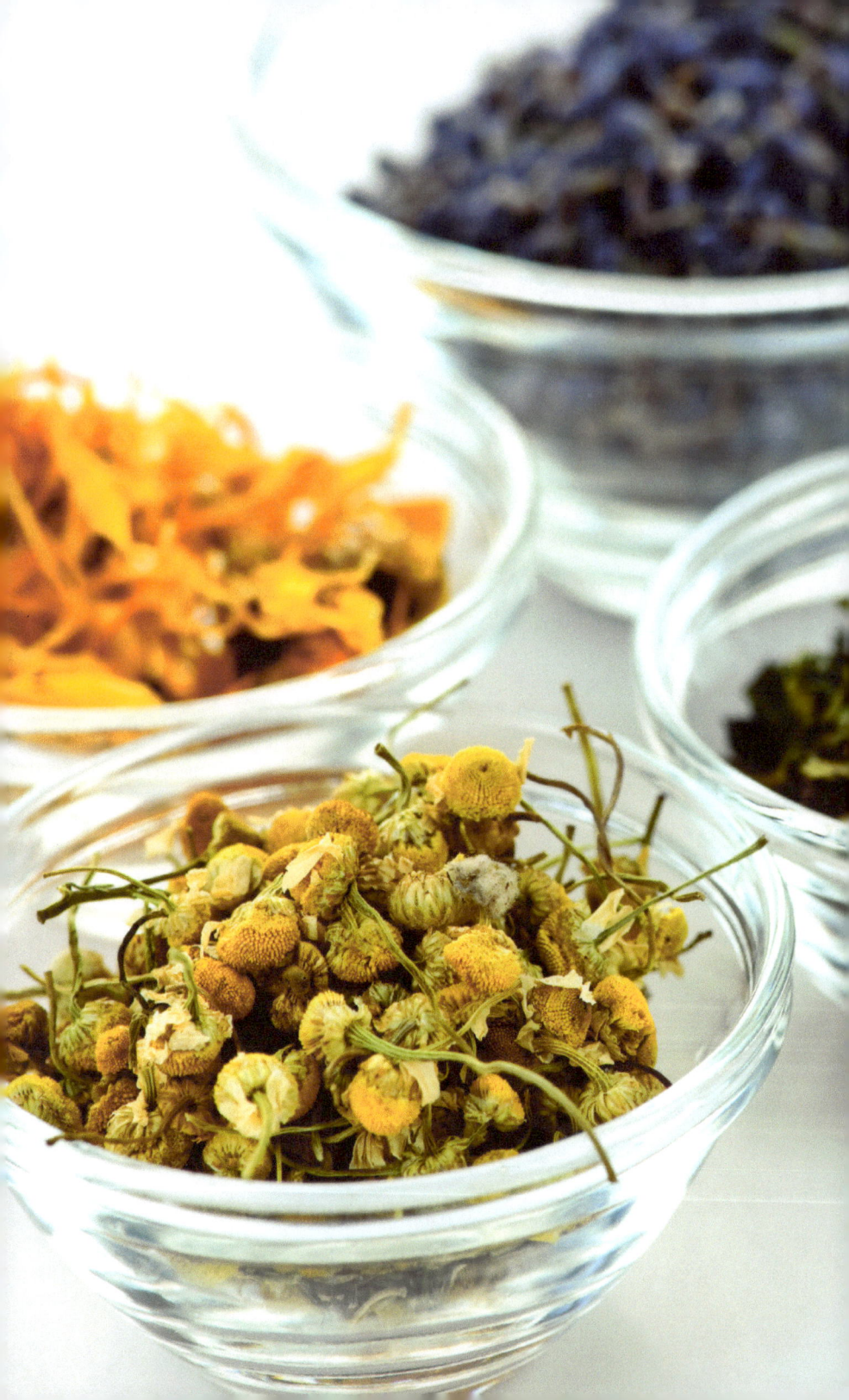

THE NATURAL ECZEMA SOLUTION:
Simple Healing Guidelines for Beautiful Skin

Copyright © 2016 Safiya Hassan

Publisher: Safiya Hassan
Editor: Christina Morgan
Designer: Angela Lockhart for Visual Communications, Inc.

The content and recipes outlined in The Natural Eczema Solution - Simple Healing Guidelines for Beautiful Skin are not intended to replace medical advice. Before using any of these treatment options it is recommended that you test a small area first. The author and publisher accept no liability with regard to the use of recipes, tecniques or guidelines in this book.

DEDICATION

This book is dedicated to my children: Hassan, Hafiz, Shayaa, Samiyra, and Taariq. I followed my passion with the hope that I may inspire you to do the same.

Believe and act as if it were impossible to fail.
    Charles F. Kettering.

ACKNOWLEDGEMENTS

A most heartfelt thank you to Ricardo Parker for his dedication to my vision and for providing graphic, design and branding development; Angela Lockhart for an amazing website design and brand development; Christina Morgan, for her direction and insight; my coach, Lalji Selassie, for his guidance; Barbara Ballard for her support and dedication to entrepreneurs and artists worldwide and Julia Chance for her valued input and contributions.

Special thanks to my mom, who is the embodiment of beauty, strength, and grace and my dad, who planted the seed of entrepreneurialism in me. Last but certainly, not least thank you to my children, who motivate me to be the best I can be every day. To Shakir Beyah for his endless support of me and my dreams.

ISBN#-13: 978-0692761342

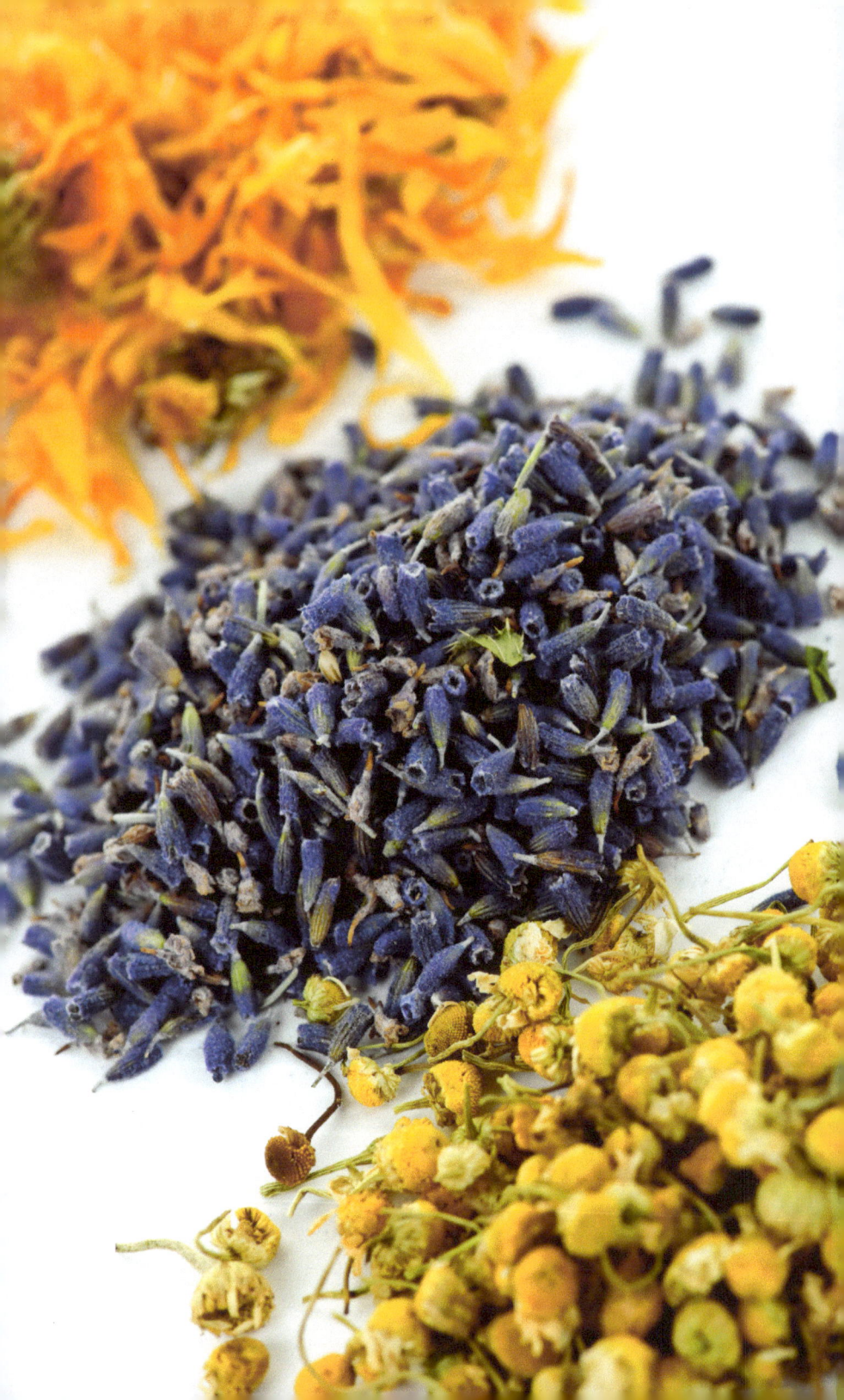

contents

FOREWARD

Letter from the first doctor to prescribe
N-Diya Healing Butter to a patient.

"A premature infant, born at thirty-four weeks, had a protracted stay in the hospital for medical reasons. During her stay I noted that she had thick, leathery skin, which over time became very scaly and friable. There was severe involvement of the scalp. At one stage it got so bad that any contact with rubbing alcohol caused the skin to bleed. As a result of the friability of the skin, a central line site became infected and the line had to be removed. At this time Aquaphor was being applied after her baths. Over time this did not seem to help.

After we used N-diya Healing Butter, there was a significant change in her skin. The skin lost its leathery appearance ; the scaling resolved, and the skin became smooth and soft. I think this product did wonders for her skin and hope it will continue to work well for her. I would strongly recommend N-diya Healing Butter for anyone with eczema.

Sincerely,
Madhu Gudavalli MD
Director of Neonatology, New York Methodist Hospital
506 Sixth Street, Brooklyn, NY 11215

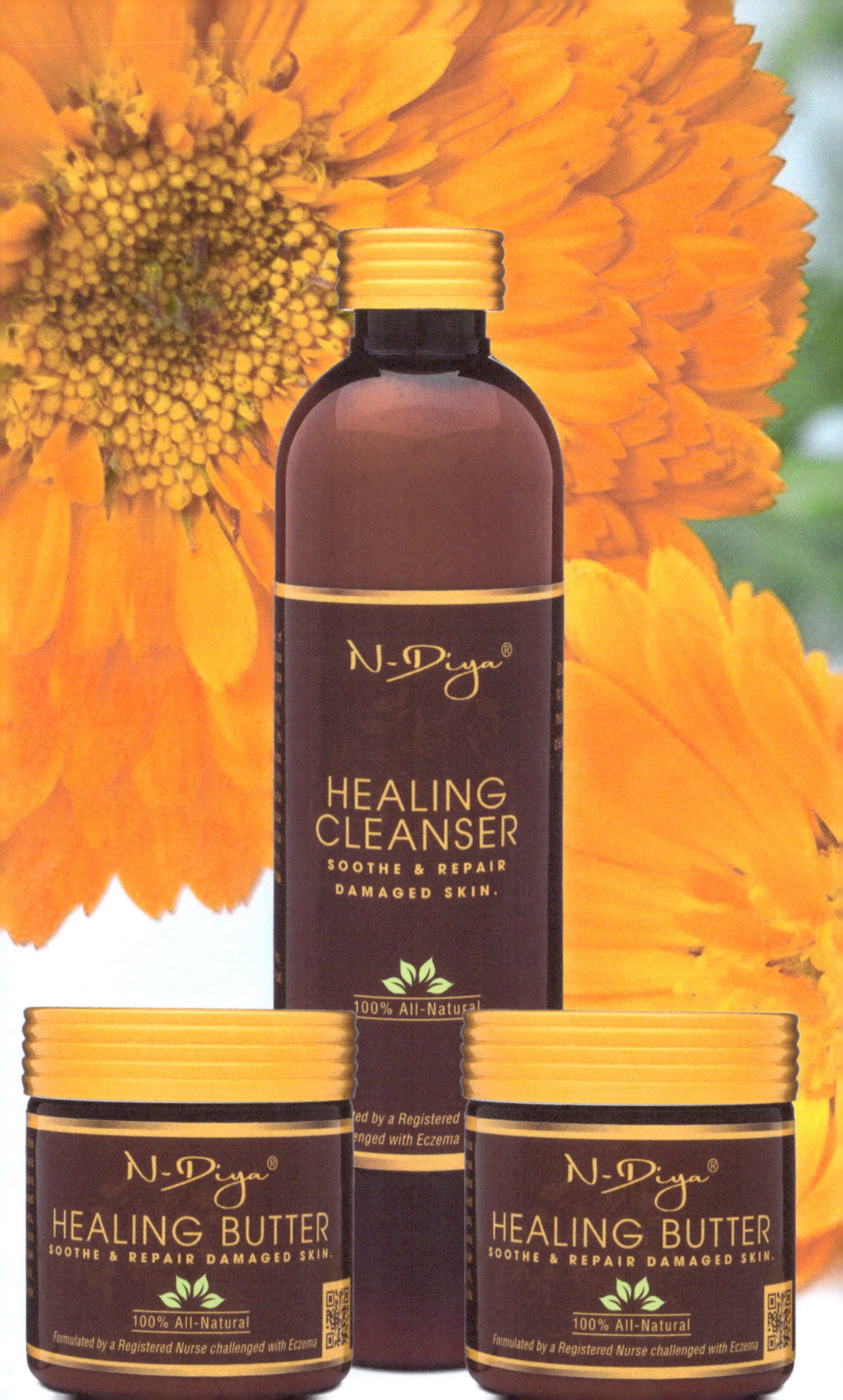

what is
eczema?

1

me and
my eczema

" I have suffered with eczema through-out my life. My first eczema-related memory is of my mother screaming: "Stop Scratching!" I still cringe a bit at the thought, but now I have to laugh because I remember all the sneaky little things I would do to relieve that incredible itch. But it was hardly a laughing matter. It was almost impossible to stop scratching even when I could see the damage I was doing to my skin, because it felt so good... initially. Regrettably, I would sometimes scratch until I bled.

My mother took me to several dermatologists where I was prescribed various topical corticosteroids. They all worked at first, but eventually my eczema would flare up again. It was a never-ending cycle.

Even as I got older I continued to have occasional episodes. Later I would learn how dangerous the excessive use of steroid creams could be."

Eczema, also referred to as atopic dermatitis, is a chronic condition that is characterized by itchy, cracked, dry and red or darkened skin depending upon your complexion. The appearance of eczema will range in severity from a mild dry patch to volcanic like eruptions. People with atopic dermatitis usually have family members who have eczema, asthma, or allergies. It affects both males and females equally, usually presents itself before the age of five and has no ethnic association.

Eczema affects approximately thirty-five million people in the United States alone, and this number is steadily rising. Medical researchers suspect this increase is directly related to the increased exposure to environmental irritants.

Simply put, eczema is the inflammation of the outer layer of the skin. But perhaps it's not so simple. Inflammation is part of a complex biological response to harmful stimuli be it a pathogen, irritant, or trauma. It is the body's way of protecting itself. Inflammation is a crucial component of the immune response and plays a very important role in the healing process.

The process of inflammation begins as the body attempts to defend itself from an irritant. Normally, inflammation endures for a period of time and resolves once the threat is reconciled. Unfortunately in the case of someone who has eczema the mechanism stays "turned on" causing damage to the tissues resulting in an insatiable itch and "the rash".

what causes
eczema?

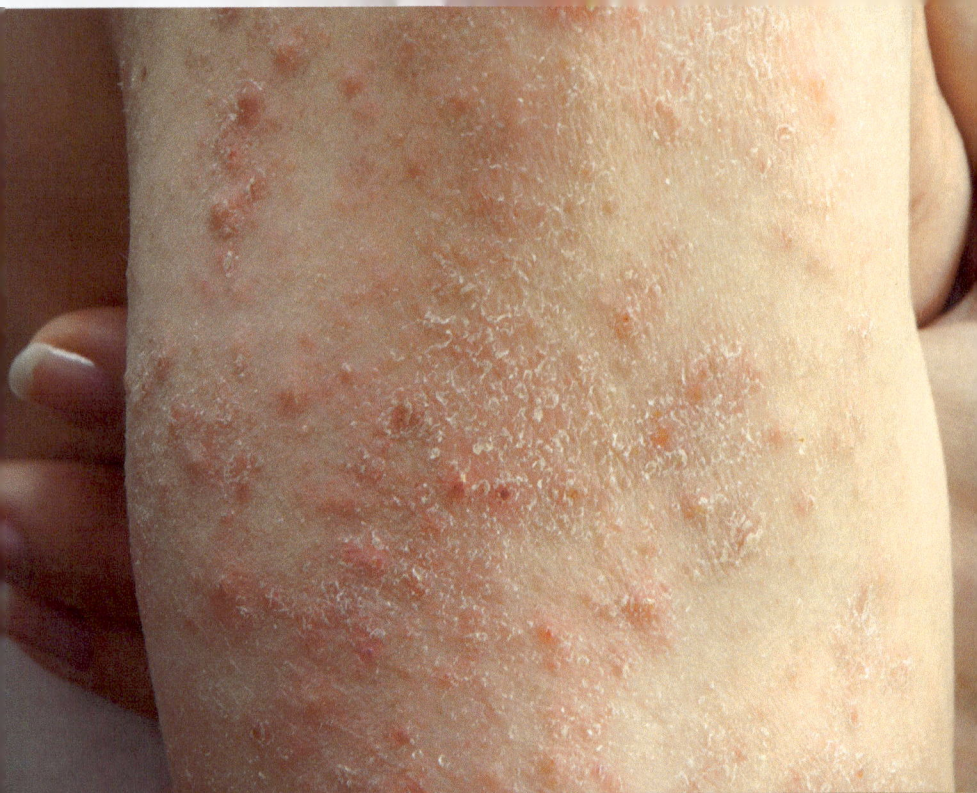

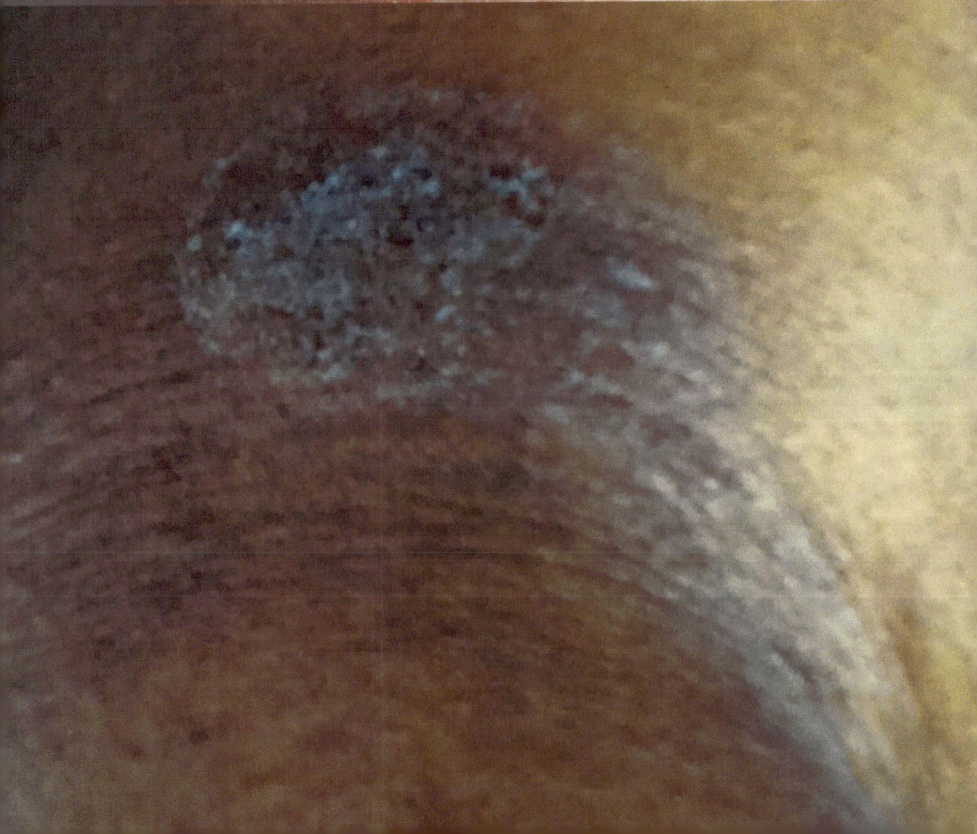

The exact cause is unknown. However, it is thought to be a combination of genetic and environmental factors. People with Eczema have an alteration in their genetic makeup that results in an increased sensitivity of their skin and a decreased ability of their skin to act as a barrier against environmental irritants.

what comes first, the itch or the rash?

3

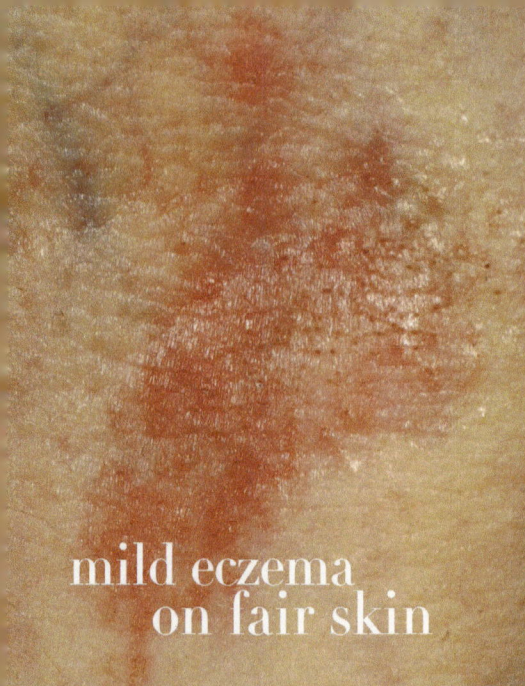

mild eczema
on fair skin

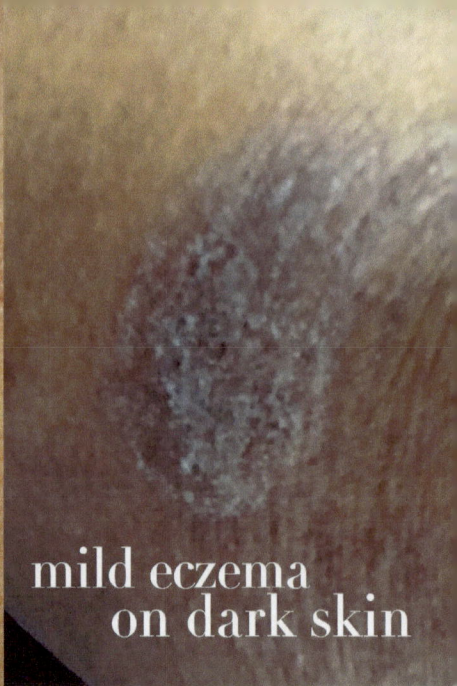

mild eczema
on dark skin

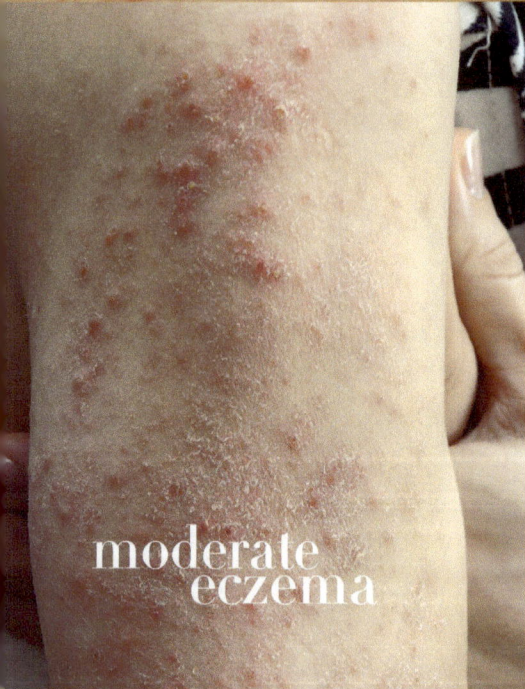

moderate
eczema

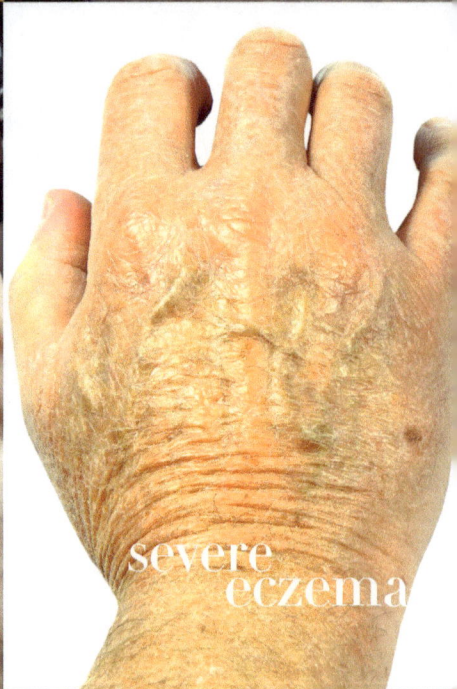

severe
eczema

The term Eczema is derived from the Greek word ekzema, which means to boil over. Anyone who has suffered from severe flare-ups knows that this best describes the appearance of the painful blisters that often burst and ooze out an unsettling fluid.

For most people it starts with a mild urge to scratch. It is seemingly harmless at first. So you scratch a little, get relief and then forget all about it. Then the urge to scratch increases. Eventually, continued scratching will result in the appearance of the rash.

Sometimes the rash doesn't appear until two to three days after contact with a trigger so it is often challenging to remember what caused that initial itchy sensation. Was it something you ate? Or was it a substance you came in contact with?

The rash of eczema varies in appearance on each person. Nevertheless, all eczema sufferers experience that same intense itching. It is the scratching done in an attempt to relieve the itch that spreads the rash and results in a worsening of the condition. Since there is no cure for eczema, affected people may experience flare-ups followed by periods of being symptom free throughout their life. Consequently, it's not an overstatement to say eczema can control every aspect of your daily existence.

standard
treatments

4

my experience with
steroid creams

During my third pregnancy, I had a flare up. I was using shea butter, which usually works for a mild flare up, but this one was severe. I was trying to avoid using steroids, but it got progressively worse and it was very unsightly and painful. Reluctantly; shortly after I delivered, I went to a dermatologist who prescribed an high-dose steroid cream.

The itching was so intense I could not wait to apply the medicine. I opened the tube on the bus ride home and began to rub it into my hand. Almost immediately, I felt an extreme burning sensation. It was so painful I wanted to scream. I actually watched the skin on my hand transform into this thin, bubbling, swelling, oozing mess. I thought if I touched it, It would just slough off. Hysterical, I began to read the pamphlet that came with the medication. The section pertaining to the side effects had a long list of life-altering effects, but the one that concerned me the most:
Caution: Do not take if you are pregnant or breastfeeding.

I was nursing at the time, so naturally this was upsetting to me beacuase had the doctor taken the time to conduct a thorough intake he would have known that the medication was contraindicated. This harrowing incident inspired me to explore my passion for alternative healing practices and led to the development of N-Diya Healing Butter to relieve my eczema.

Severe Eczema can result in a decreased quality of life for the suffer. But there is light at the end of the tunnel. You can have the beautiful skin you deserve by following the simple guidelines in this book.

A common treatment for eczema is topical corticosteroids. This is a steroid in the form of a cream that you apply directly to the skin. They are categorized as anti-inflammatories. Corticosteroids are an effective short-term treatment for eczema. They work by inhibiting the inflammatory response. While they temporarily suppress the signs and symptoms of eczema they do not cure the underlining condition. The problem with using corticosteroids is that you can develop a dependency on them with continual use. You will begin to require higher doses to get the same relief you once were able to achieve at lower doses. It is important to note that there are side effects ranging from mild to life threatening and that the risks of experiencing these side effects increase with prolonged use and increased dosage.

Oral or injectable forms of this drug are only used as a last resort as side effects and risks are even greater.

side effects
can include:

TACHYPHYLAXIS	This is a tolerence or dependency that can occur after prolong use
HYPERGLYCEMIA	Increase blood glucose level
CUSING SYNDROME	Complex systemic imbalance caused by excessive exposure to hormones
HYPOTHAIAMIC	Pituitary axis supression
SUPER INFECTION	Due to supression of the immune system
TELANGIECTASIA	Distended blood vessels
STRIAE *(stretch marks)*	Resulting from the loss of collagen and elastin in the skin
SKIN ATROPHY	Dry, thin fragile skin
MACERATION	Softening and breaking down of the skin
CATARACTS	Found with high dose and long term use when applied around the eyes
GLAUCOMA	Usually expereience when ointments are applied around the eyes or it is taken systemically
GASTRO-INTESTINAL EFFECTS	Nausea, vomiting and peptic ulcers.

GROWTH RETARDATION IN CHILDREN

TOPICAL STEROID ADDICTION
Also referred to as Steroid Withdrawal Syndrome (See page to the right)

Category C Pregnancy - Corticosteroids are teratogenic in laboratory animals. There are no studies on pregnant women but it is recommended that pregnant women and nursing mothers avoid corticosteroids to avoid potential risk to the fetus and newborn.

topical steroid addiction.

Recent attention to studies linking the prolonged use of steroid creams to a condition called Topical Steroid Addiction (TSA) aka Steroid Withdrawal Syndrome, have led to the re-evaluation of using corticosteroids to treat eczema. TSA often begins with the development of a tolerence to the steroids being administered. The initial dose no longer produces the desired effect so stronger doses are prescribed. The body eventually becomes dependent on this "chemical" to maintain homeostasis. When you abruptly cease taking the medication you will experience a super inflammation of the skin or a rebound effect. At this point the flare up is not a result of contact with a trigger, it is now caused by the withdrawal of the medication. These flare ups are usually more severe and difficult to control.

If you have been using topical corticosteroids beyond the recommended safety period of two weeks or more and have noticed your flare-ups seem to be getting worse and requiring stronger doses with each episode, you may be addicted to steroids. If you think this is a possibility, seek a dermatologist familiar with this condition that can make the proper diagnosis and assist you with the withdrawal process.

trial, error breakthrough!

my breakthrough!

I have always been fascinated by the healing properties in natural resources - herbs, flowers and roots. I'd listen in awe to my elders talk about how they used herbal remedies to treat specific ailments. As an adult, I became a registered nurse, but natural remedies and natural healing modalities continued to intrigue me. After several trips to the dermatologist and leaving with a stronger dose of steroids each time, I began to experience new side effects including immediate burning and the deterioration of my skin. It was then that I decided I would find another solution to my problem. I began to research and study the medicinal properties of herbs, essential oils, and botanicals.

I combined this knowledge with my nursing experience to formulate N-diya, a line of therapeutic products created from some of the most powerful healing agents in nature. I don't know how many batches I threw out before I was satisfied! But I knew that the end product had to yield the satisfactory results I was looking for.

The skin-care needs of someone with eczema are challenging. My product had to:

- *Moisturize my severely dry skin without leaving a greasy film.*
- *Soothe the insane itching*
- *Reduce inflammation and swelling*
- *Soften my rough, thickened skin*
- *Restore my complexion*

Basically, I needed something that would make my skin beautiful again. When I finally got it right, I was ecstatic. The first time someone commented on how soft and smooth my skin felt, it was music to my ears.

While I'm happy my products worked so well to soothe symptoms, the primary goal is to avoid flare-ups in the first place. The Natural Eczema Solution contains the information you need to understand and get in control of your eczema so you can live your life to the fullest.

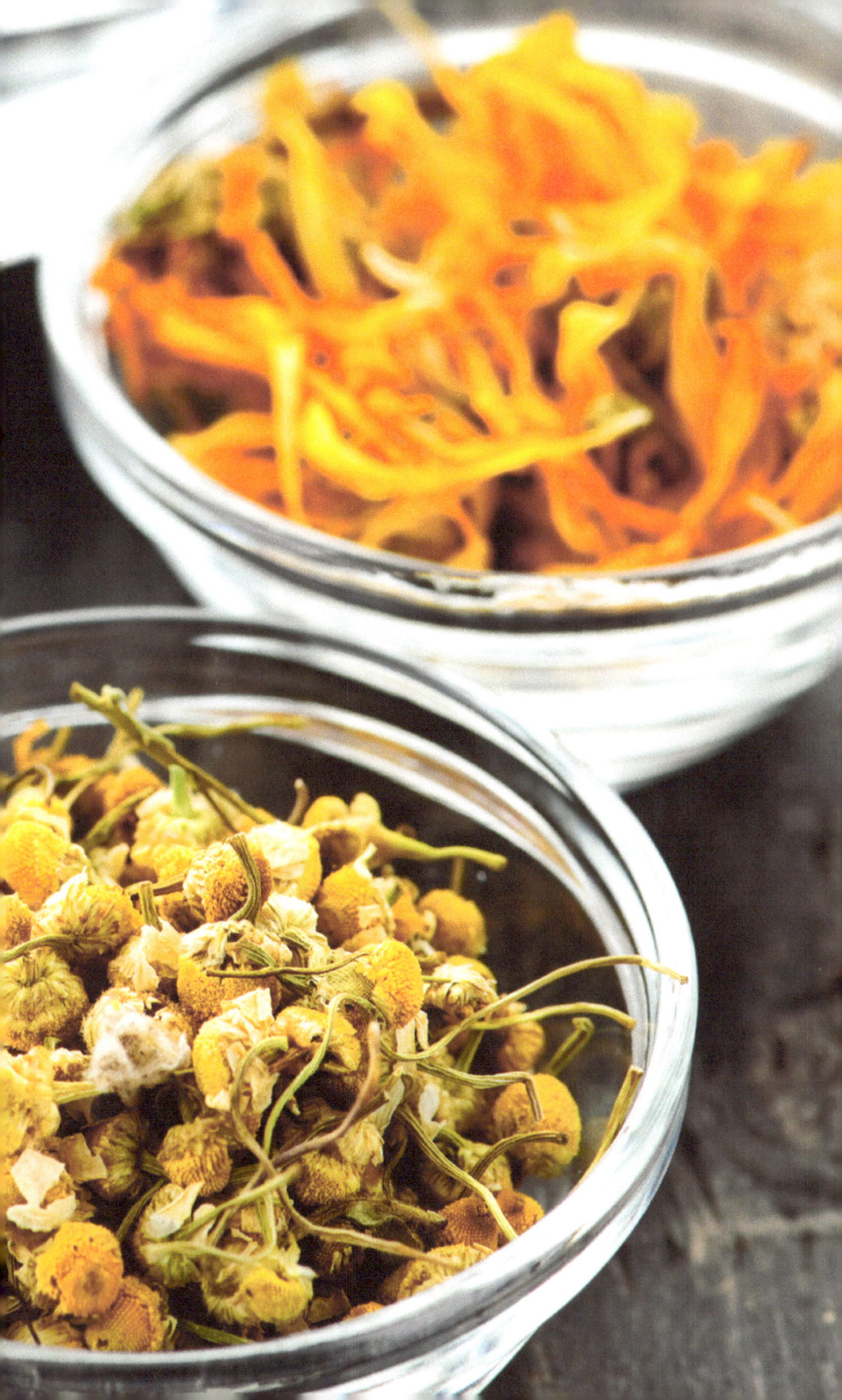

discovering.
your triggers

Optimal physical and mental health are key in managing eczema. Your primary course of action, however, is to identify your triggers so that you can avoid flare-ups. Otherwise, no matter what you use as a treatment, you will not see a complete resolution. For example, your eczema treatments will not be effective if tomatoes are your trigger, and you continue to eat them. You must do your best to avoid contact with your triggers at all times.

It will require some level of discipline and maybe some lifestyle changes to care for your sensitive skin. You must begin to read ingredient labels on your food, personal care products, household cleansers, etc., in order to avoid triggers.

"Unfortunately I learned the hard way. After multiple flare-ups I realized that when I was exposed to harsh detergents or cleansers, my skin would become irritated and itchy. Stress was another cause of severe flare-ups for me."

The best way to determine what is causing your outbreaks is to see an allergist. To find a licensed professional allergist near you ask your primary physican for a referral.

If you cannot see an allergist, it's a good idea to eliminate all known triggers and reintroduce them one at a time to gauge your response. Keep a diary to track your daily meals and contact with new substances (such as a new body wash) for approximately three to six months. This will help you identify your triggers through process of elimination and reintroduction.

harsh soaps
(e.g., laundry detergents, shampoos, dish detergents)

fragrances

synthetic or rough fabrics

dairy products

eggs

nuts

soy products

wheat

shell fish

chemicals
(e.g., bleach)

cigarette smoke

pollen

pet dander

dust mites

molds

extreme heat

extreme cold

high humidity

low humidity

stress

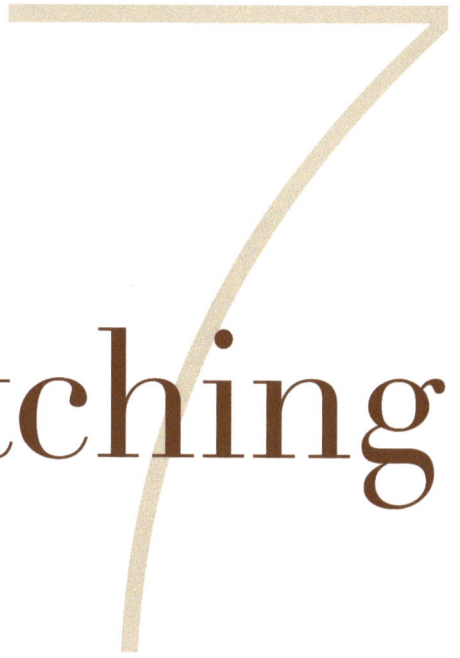

stop
scratching

7

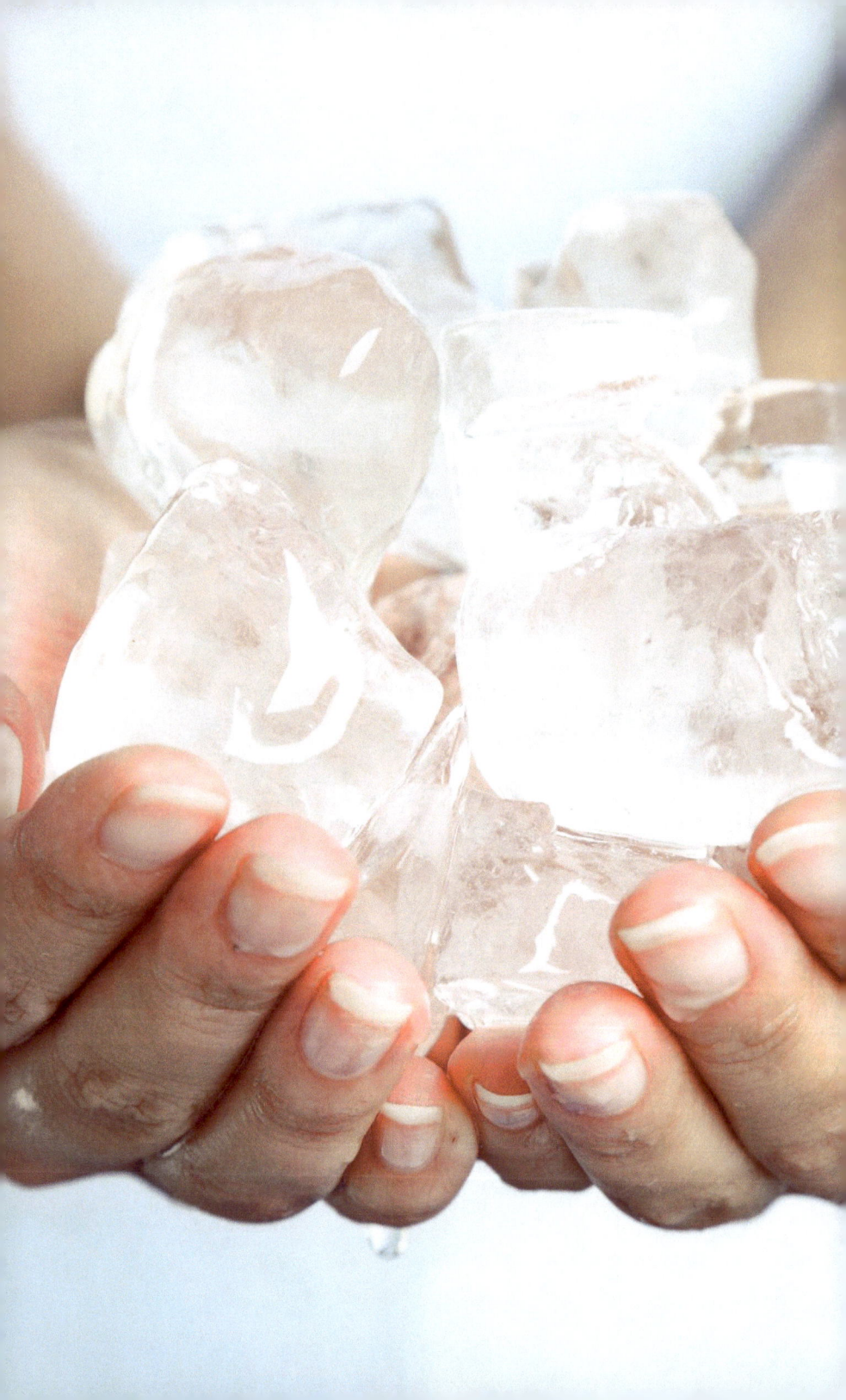

"stop scratching,

Ok, I should be the last person to tell you
not to scratch.
I of all people, know how incredibly difficult it is, but it is key
to managing your eczema flare ups. "

Scratching will spread the rash and lead to open sores and scarring. Keeping your skin well moisturized will help soothe a mild itch. For severe flare-ups, look for emollients that have soothing herbs and botanicals to soothe and heal your dry, itchy skin. (e.g., N-diya Healing Butter)

tips

- Avoid rough fabrics

- Keep nails short and clean to lessen damage when you do give in

- Place a cold compress at the site of the itch to provide some relief

- Keep skin clean and moisturized

- Be aware of habitual scratching e.g., scratching when stressed, tired or bored

- Try to focus on something else

how does stress trigger
eczema?

8

me stress and eczema

My stress-induced flare-ups were the most vicous because they were not localized. Whenever I experienced a flare-up resulting from contact with a chemical it was confined to the affected area, spreading only after I scratched. But when I was stressed the itching just seem to erupt anywhere and everywhere making it more difficult to manage.

The stress response is an automatic reflex to events that make us feel threatened or uncomfortable. When you sense danger, real or imagined, your body responds by going into "fight or flight" mode and begins to systematically prepare you to cope with the event at hand by:

- Increasing the heart rate, blood pressure, and respiration.

- Restricting blood flow from functions like digestion and tissue perfusion.

- Redirecting blood flow to the heart and large muscles.

- Releasing hormones like adrenaline and cortisol into the bloodstream.

- Releasing stored glucose.

This process is why in extreme emergencies people can experience superhuman strength to do things they wouldn't ordinarily be able to do. A great example of this is having the ability to lift a car off of someone in a moment of panic. Typically this transformation is harmless because the body reverts back to its normal state after the event. The problem occurs when you remain at this heightened state for prolonged periods of time due to life events like exams, relationship issues, challenges at work, traffic jams, or unpaid bills.

Granted, these modern stressors are not the same as being attacked by a bear, but our body responds in the same manner. Anxiety can trigger a moderate stress response, but unlike the quick resolution of a bear attack - escape or die! - you can worry about an unpaid bill for days, resulting in a build up of hormones that can wreak havoc on the body when found in excessive amounts.

consistent high
stress level can result in

- Cardiovascular disease

- High blood pressure

- Susceptibility to infection

- Skin eruptions

- Pain

- Diabetes

- Infertility

During the stress response, blood is redirected from normal daily functions like tissue perfusion to prepare the body to "fight or flight". This redirection results in a decrease in blood circulation to the skin, further weakening the skin barrier and potentially hindering normal healing. For someone who has eczema, this would be the ultimate insult to his or her already dry, itchy, damaged and fragile skin.

Ironically, stress triggers your eczema or makes an existing flare-up worst and having a flare-up is stressful. This can create a vicious cycle. It may seem impossible to break this cycle but, you can take steps to reduce your stress by establishing a wellness regimen.

finding your own coping mechanisms

1. First, identify and eliminate the causes of stress in your life. If they can't be eliminated, decide how you will limit your exposure to stressors, or change how you think and react to them.

2. Second, participate in activities that will improve your mood and make you feel good. Take time out for yourself and identify what works for you, be it a relaxing bath, a massage, meditation, or yoga.

3. Third, the power of positive thinking will go a long way in seeing you through the challenges you will face in life, including eczema. The power is in your thought process.

Let's examine the following scenario:

getting fired

Subject #1 - Thinks of all the bills that have to be paid and the daily expenses of life. Focuses on all the media coverage of the failing economy, the people he knows that have been unsuccessful in finding a job and believes that he will too experience difficulty getting a job. After thinking about all the has gone wrong and will go wrong, he can see no way out of his despair.

Subject #2 - Thinks of how he was never completely happy at his job and sees this as an opportunity to explore his passions and to earn an income doing something fulfilling that he loves. He applies for unemployment, creates a tighter budget, and cuts back on all excessive spending. He enrolls in school to gain further knowledge of his new career goal and decides that getting fired was truly a blessing.

One event, two different responses. Both subjects have the ability to choose how to react. The anxiety level of subject #1 will be higher as a result of his thought pattern. Your mind is your most powerful tool in managing your stress. How you think will determine whether or not you set off your stress response. It is unrealistic to think you will avoid stress altogether. However, your ability to control how you react is key to managing eczema.

Don't let eczema become the focal point of your life. While you're trying to keep it under control, it is very easy for it to overwhelm you and become a great source of stress. Remember, the goal is to live a very full life with as few interruptions from eczema as possible.

psychological effects of having a
skin condition.

eczema's
pyschological impact

" I often experienced severe flare-ups that resulted in thick leathery, dry, cracked and darkened skin. I remember the lengths I would go to in order to avoid awkward situations and the mean things people would say about my rashes. It was challenging to develop self-esteem as a young person. I remember overhearing many unkind remarks about my skin that made me want to cry, and sometimes I did. I think what made it easier for me was shifting my attention away from my eczema to doing activities that I loved. Eventually, I began to develop my inner qualities like kindness, generosity and self determination and I began to feel good about myself. I loved to dance so I took ballet, jazz, tap, modern, and African dance. Eczema was the last thing on my mind when I was in the middle of the dance floor! This fostered a strong sense of self that was independent of my outward appearance. It helped me to believe in my abilities and in myself. Eventually, I developed "thick" skin, pun intended, and I began to care less about what people thought of me.

I would be lying if I said I never questioned why eczema afflicted me. I remember asking, "Lord, why me? Why is my skin so ugly?" But now I am grateful. I believe having eczema has made it easier for me to march to the beat of my own drum. There's a certain freedom that comes from not caring what people think of you. Having eczema was a blessing for me. It motivated me to formulate a line of skin and hair care products, start my own company, and write this book.

Developing self-confidence is a challenge when your physical appearance is altered. During an eczema flare-up your skin is delicate and fragile.

Constant scratching can lead to scarring, open sores, discoloration, and thickening of the skin.

You start expending a great deal of energy trying to hide your rash, and you can become self-conscious to the point that you avoid social activities and interactions.

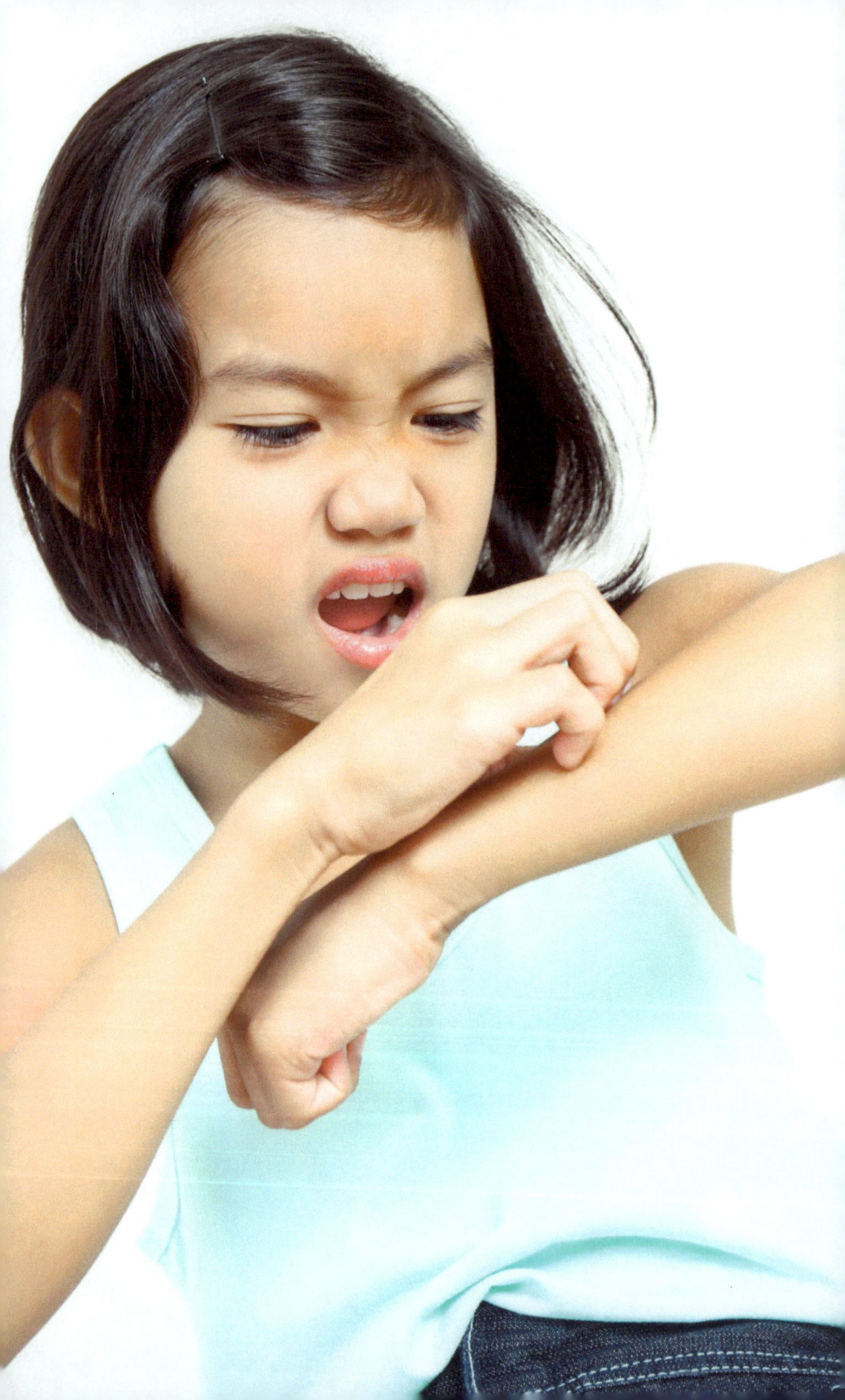

10

children and eczema

We all know the saying: kids can be cruel. Coping with visible ailments is especially difficult for children and teenagers when bullying and teasing is involved, but parents can help. Encourage your child to discover their passion and develop their talents. It will make them feel good about themselves and help them to build self confidence.

Tell them that they are beautiful or handsome, but focus more on their inner qualities and achievements. Your compliments should place a value on who they are and not what they look like. How you look on the outside will change throughout your life. Confidence tied to your inner value is lasting.

Watch out for signs that your child is withdrawing and becoming stressed and/or depressed. The following are loose guidelines for what to look out for; but you know your child best, and it is a good idea to seek help if you have any concerns about their mental and emotional health.

chart signs
of distress
that require clinical treatment

emotional signs of depression	• Constant sadness
	• Irritability
	• Hopelessness
	• Feeling worthless or guilty for no reason
	• Loss of interest in favorite activities

physical symptoms of depression	• Trouble sleeping
	• Low energy or fatigue
	• Significant weight change
	• Difficulty concentrating

when to seek urgent help!	• Thoughts of suicide
	• Panic attacks
	• Aggressive behavior
	• Extreme anger
	• Violent behavior

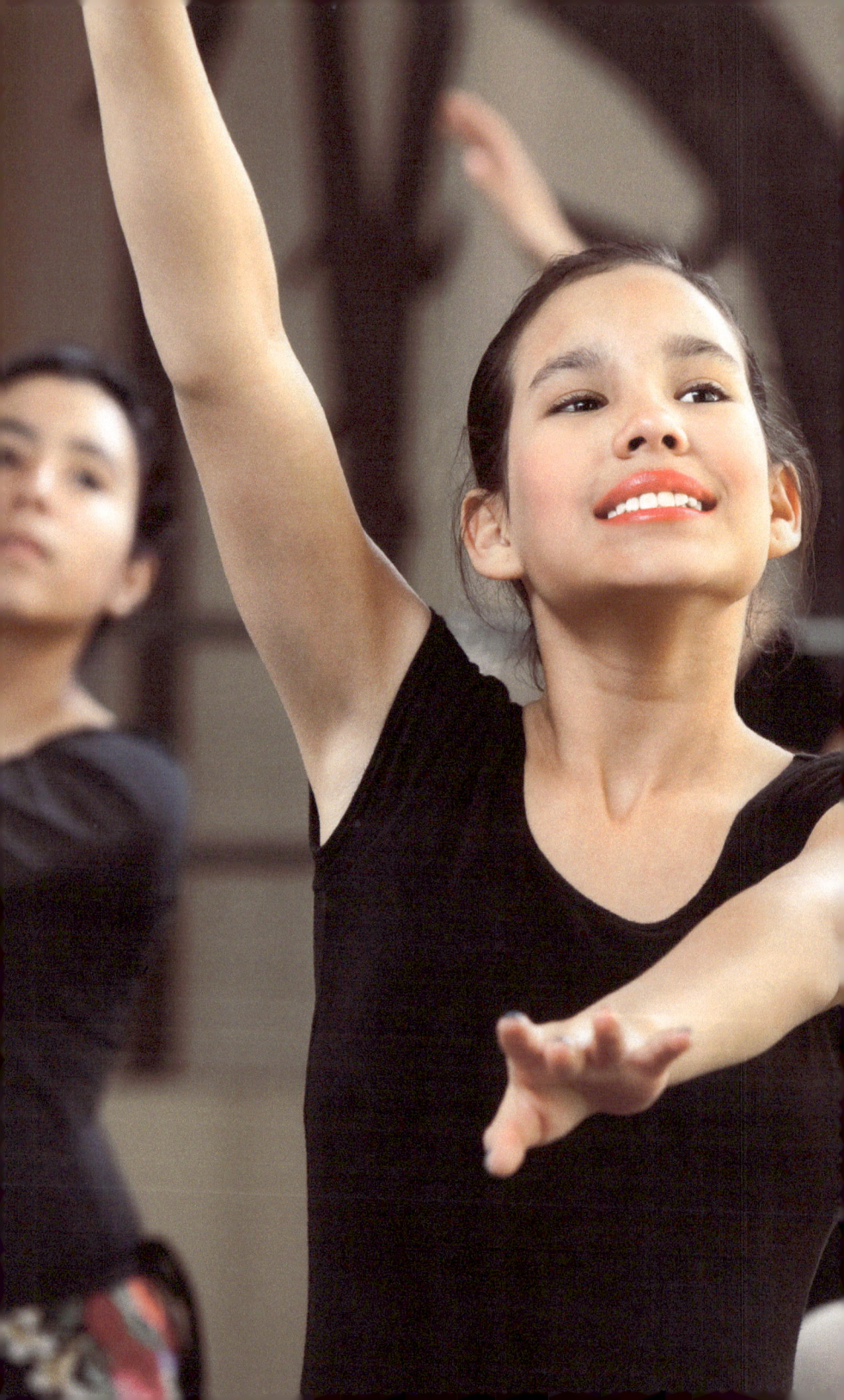

if your child
has eczema,
help them to develop a healthy sense of self by
engaging in sports, dance, art
or any activity
that they are interested in.
Accomplishments will help them
feel good
about themselves
and take the focus off of their
skin condition.

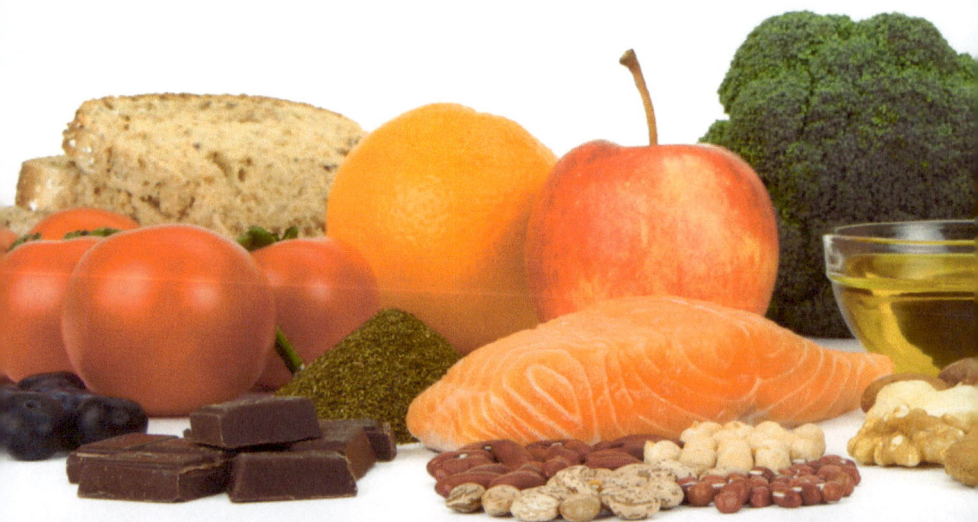

11

let food
be thy medicine

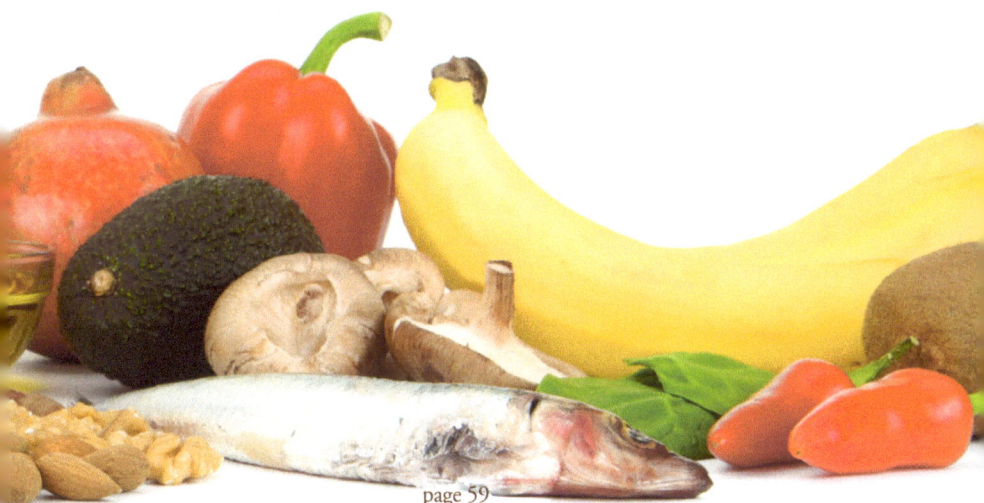

your diet
is an essential part of your
healing process.

The healthier you are, the easier it will be to manage your eczema. When you are properly nourished, your ability to ward of skin infection and repair damaged skin increases. Your body is designed to break down and distribute nutrients from whole food sources. When a large part of your diet consist of foods that are processed, pasteurized, and genetically engineered, most of the nutritional value is destroyed. To ensure adequate nutritional intake keep your food sources as close to nature as possible. This means less food from boxes and cans and more fresh fruit, vegetables and whole grains.

Organic fruit and vegetables are healthier for you but they can be more expensive. However, you don't need to purchase all your fruits and vegetables organic. Fruits like bananas and pineapples have thick skins that will be removed before consumption so you are not likely to ingest harmful pesticides. However, it is recommended that you purchase organic grapes and strawberries since the skin will not be removed before eating. Juicing fruits and vegetables is a good way of getting large amounts of nutrients into the bloodstream and into your cells. I purchased a juicer for my birthday two years ago and have been juicing consistantly ever since and I feel younger, more energetic, and my skin looks amazing. Invest in your health it is your greatest asset. The only side effect of eating healthy is feeling good and being well!

Experiment with healthy recipes. Be patient with yourself and your taste buds and you may be surprised to learn how delicious and fun eating healthy can be.

Recommended foods to purchase

organic

- celery
- pears
- peaches
- apples
- cherries
- strawberries
- grapes
- spinach
- potatoes
- bell peppers
- raspberries
- berries

enhanced

The process of healing injured skin places an increased met, healing may be hindered. Research has shown that increa vitamin C and vitamin A, can aid the healing process by scarring.

SOURCES OF PROTEIN
- Beef
- Chicken
- Fish
- Milk
- Yogurt
- Cheese

VEGETARIAN SOURCES OF PROTEIN
- Broccoli
- Spinach
- Kale
- Cauliflower
- Nuts
- Beans

SOURCES OF VITAMIN A
- Liver
- Red pepper, cayenne pepper, chili powder papprika
- Sweet potato
- Carrots
- Dark green leafy vegetables
- Butternut squash
- Dried herbs
- Dried apricots
- Cantaloupe

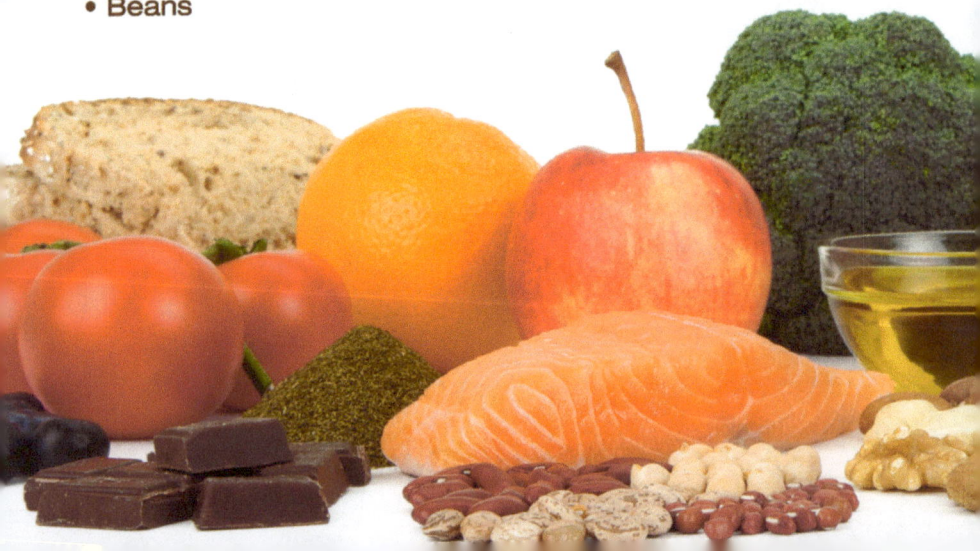

healing.

metabolic demand on the body. If these requirements are not
sing the daily-recommended servings of protein, zinc and
accelerating healing time and minimizing the chance of

SOURCES OF ZINC
- Beef
- Liver
- Crab
- Sunflower seed
- Peanut butter
- Whole grain

SOURCES OF VITAMIN C
- Guava
- Pineapples
- Papaya
- Bell Peppers
- Broccoli
- Brussel Sprouts
- Strawberries
- Oranges
- Kiwi
- Lemon

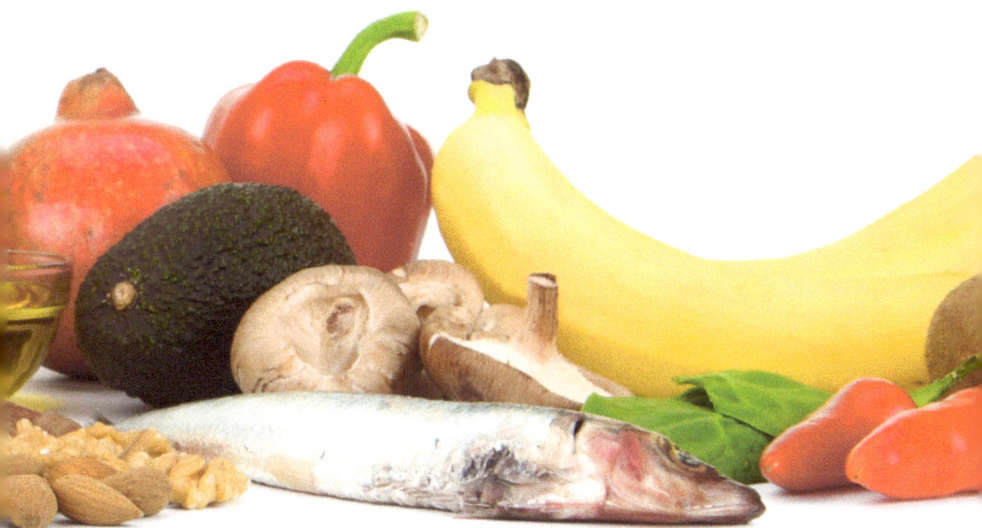

eating foods rich in
probiotics
can help alleviate
eczema

Probiotics are live bacteria and yeast that are good for your health. They maintain balance in the gastro-intestinal system and strengthen the immune system. Bacteria is present within the intestinal tract. Without the presence of probiotics to keep them in check, harmful bacteria can thrive and create disease. A study on probiotics have also proven them to be beneficial in preventing eczema in children when probiotic supplements were given to pregnant women with a family history of eczema or allergies. There is some evidence that at the very least it may reduce the severity of the disease in those who do develop eczema.

foods rich in probiotics

- plain unflavored yogurt
- kefir
- sauerkraut
- miso
- pickles
- tempeh
- kimchi
- kombucha tea
- dark chocolate
- soy milk

12

getting and staying clear

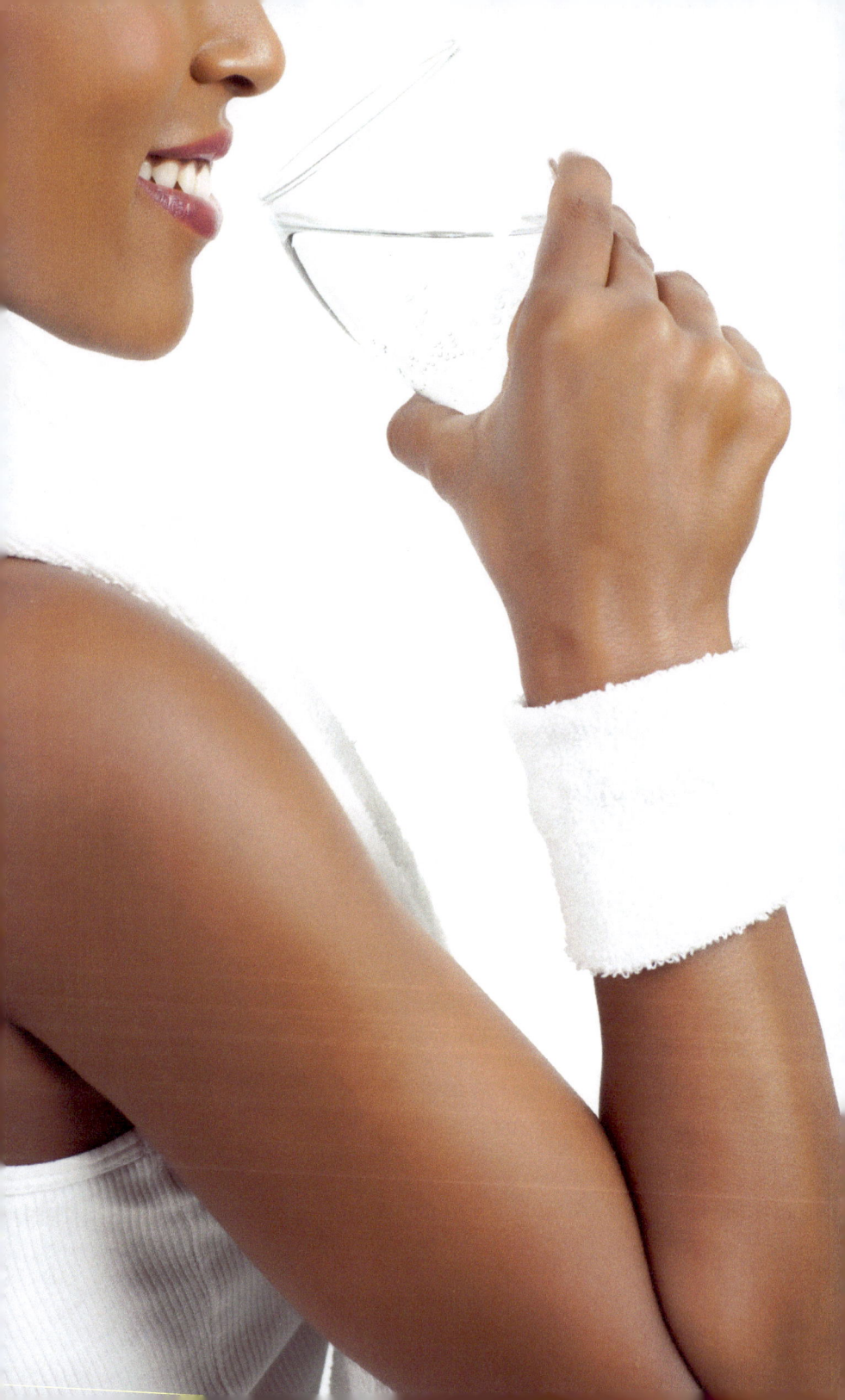

Limit your intake of substances that are diuretics. They drain fluid from the body. Drinking excessive amounts may result in dehidration and a depletion of vitamin A, which is essential for skin renewal. Dehydration can not only trigger a flare-up, they can make an existing one worse.

staying hydrated is
important!

Please consider eliminating alcohol from your diet during an outbreak or at the very least limiting your intake to prevent further irritation to your already dry and sensitive skin.

symptoms of
dehydration

- thirst & dry mouth
- fatigue
- decreased urine / dark urine
- muscle cramps
- cessation of sweat
- cessation of tears
- confusion
- weakness

13

proper waste elimination

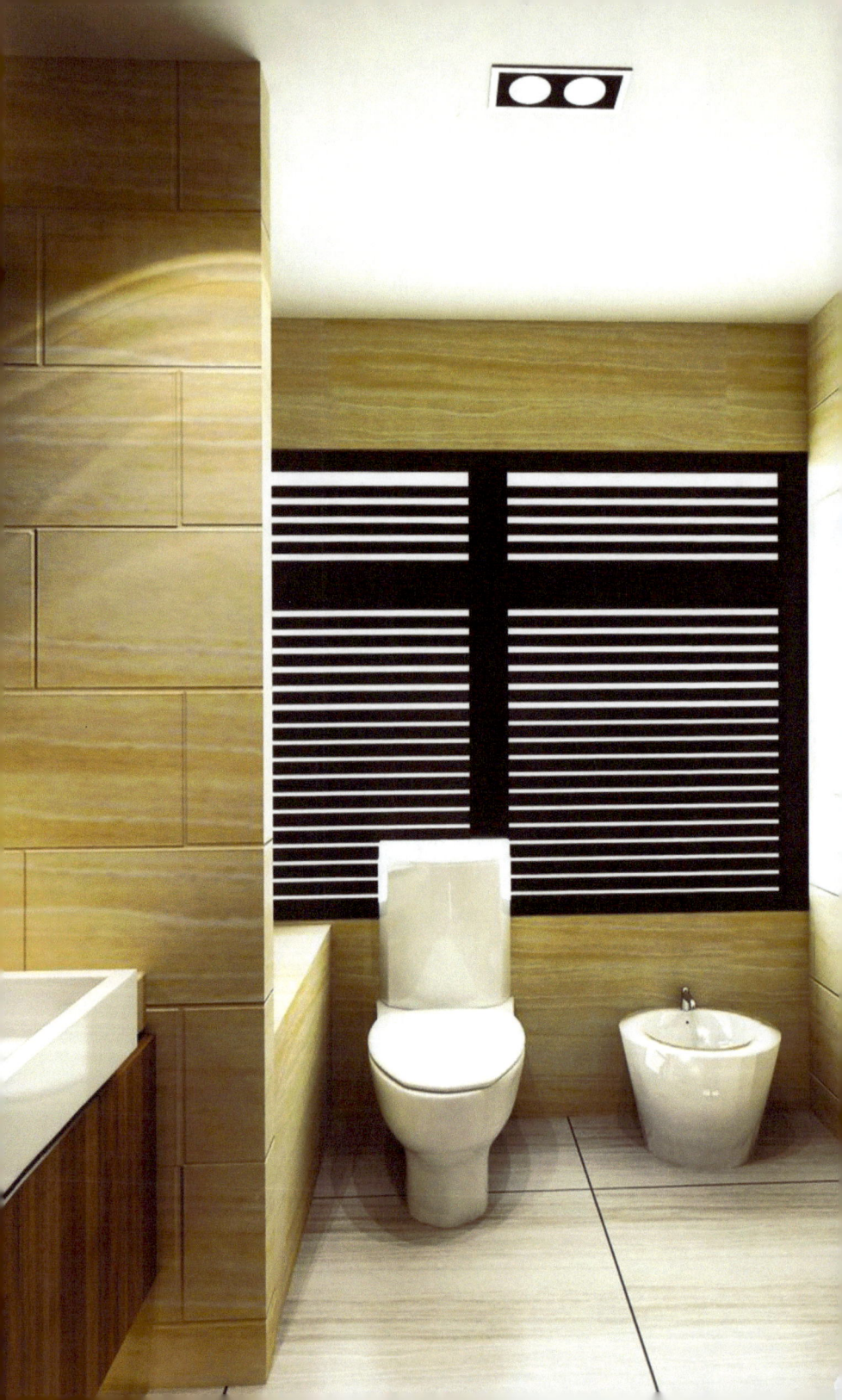

All organisms, even one-cell organisms break down food to absorb nutrients and expel waste. When your elimination system is functioning properly you empty your bowels at least two times a day with ease.

A lack of fiber in your diet, dehydration, stress, and ignoring one's natural urge to go can cause constipation. Without proper bowel function, waste that should be eliminated stays in the body rots, and decays. This leaves a gluey residue along the intestinal wall which builds up over time and the rotting fecal matter begins to produce toxins. Not a pretty picture.

A build up of toxins in the body impacts your health in general but it places extra stress on the elimination organs, including the skin.

Here are some tips to
keep your bowels regular

- Drink at least two quarts of water a day

- Eat whole foods e.g., fruits, vegetables and grains that contain fiber

- Relax

- Don't eat in a hurry

- Chew your food thoroughly as digestion begins in the mouth

- Exercise on a regular basis. It stimulates and tones intestinal muscles to facilitate proper waste elimination

- Avoid abusing laxatives. The frequent use of laxatives to resolve constipation can weaken the intestines and result in an inability to move your bowels without their assistance.

- When you have to go... ..go

14

sleep

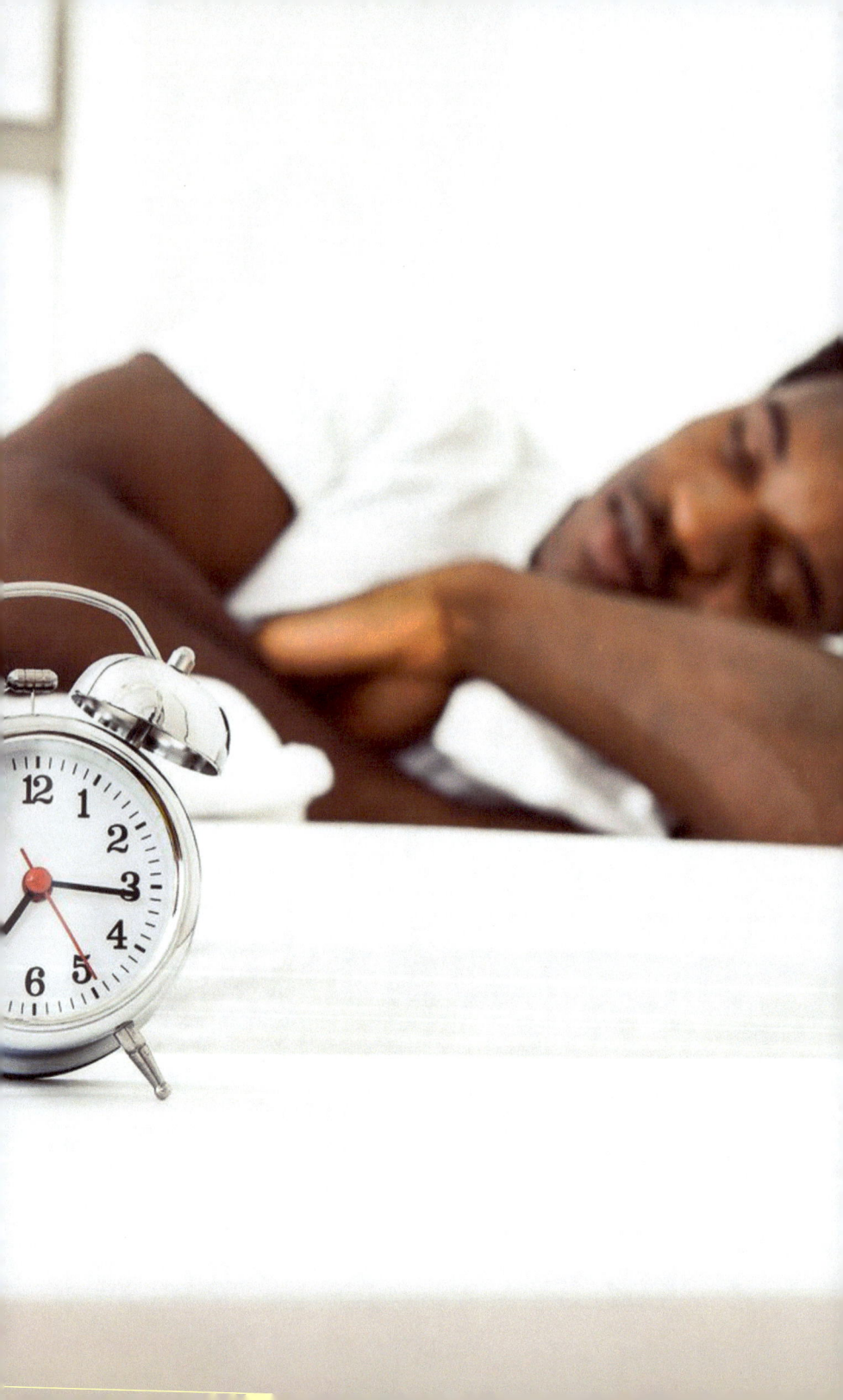

Yes, beauty sleep is very important. While you may think that you are just lying there dreaming and doing nothing, it's actually more complicated then that. Your mind and body are still at work. When you are sleep the body restores and heals itself. During the early stages of the sleep cycle, surges of growth hormones fill the body, which contributes to what people call "beauty sleep." This helps to repair and rebuild tissues and stimulate collagen formation, thus maintaining your youthful appearance.

A good night's sleep is crucial to your physical and mental health. Lack of sleep impairs the healing process, weakens the immune system, and can cause or worsen health issues. For people with eczema, a good night's sleep is crucial, because your skin repairs itself during this time. You need sleep in order for healing to take place.

age	hours of sleep
infant	14-15
toddler	12-14
school age	10-11
adults	7-9

exercise 15

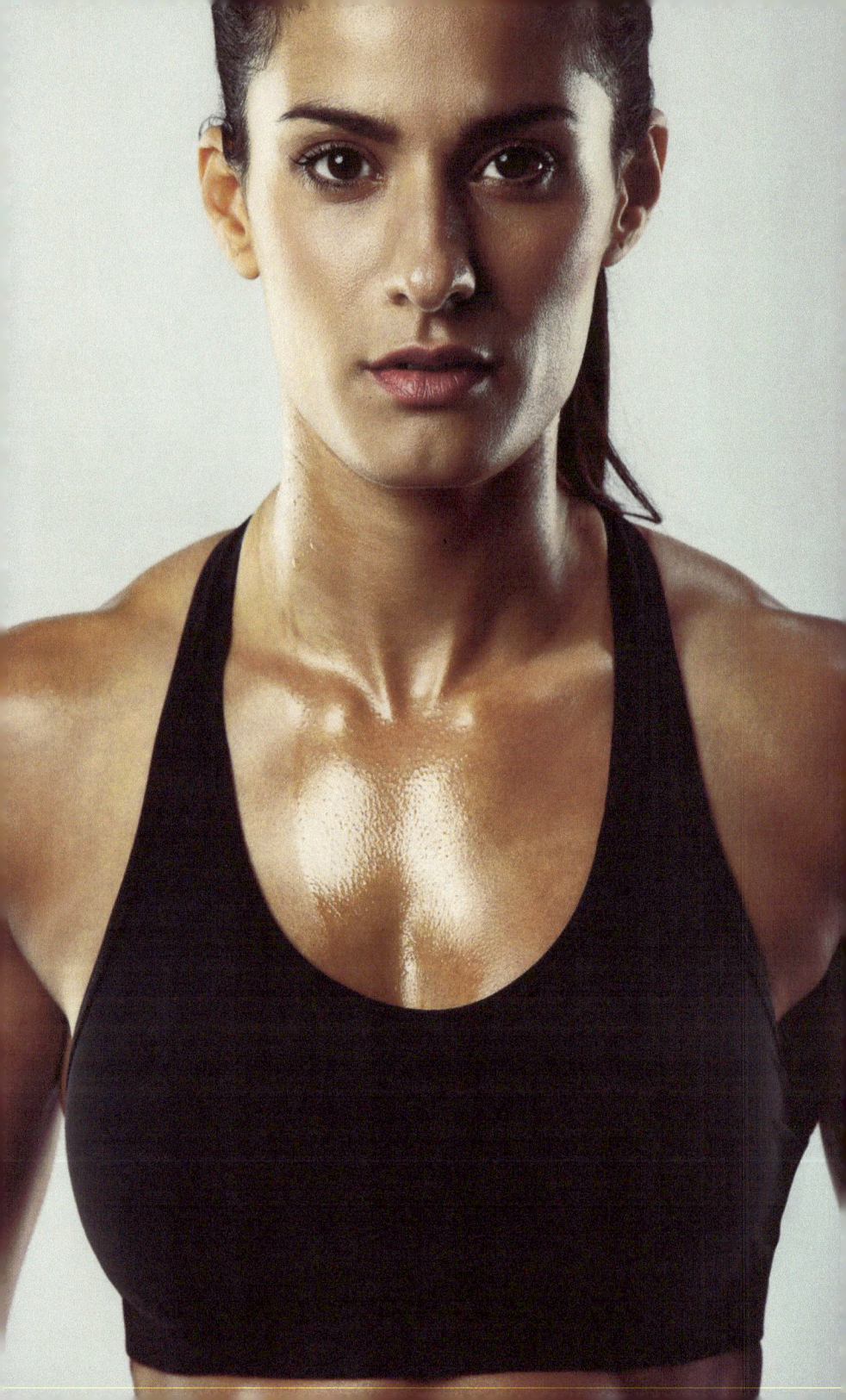

Exercise is great for improving cardiac and respiratory function. This increases your body's ability to transport nutrients and oxygen to your cells and to carry waste away from the cells. The benefit of exercise to your overall health is endless. Optimal circulation is essential for the healing process and another great benefit is healthy, glowing skin!

Exercise is also a great stress reliever and combats anxiety and depression by releasing natural feel-good chemicals like endorphins which give you a natural high.

Exercise doesn't have to be limited to working out at the gym it can be any activity that gets the heart pumping, such as walking, dancing, biking, skating, etc.

Find something that you enjoy to increase the chance you'll
stick with it.

establishing a natural skin care regimen

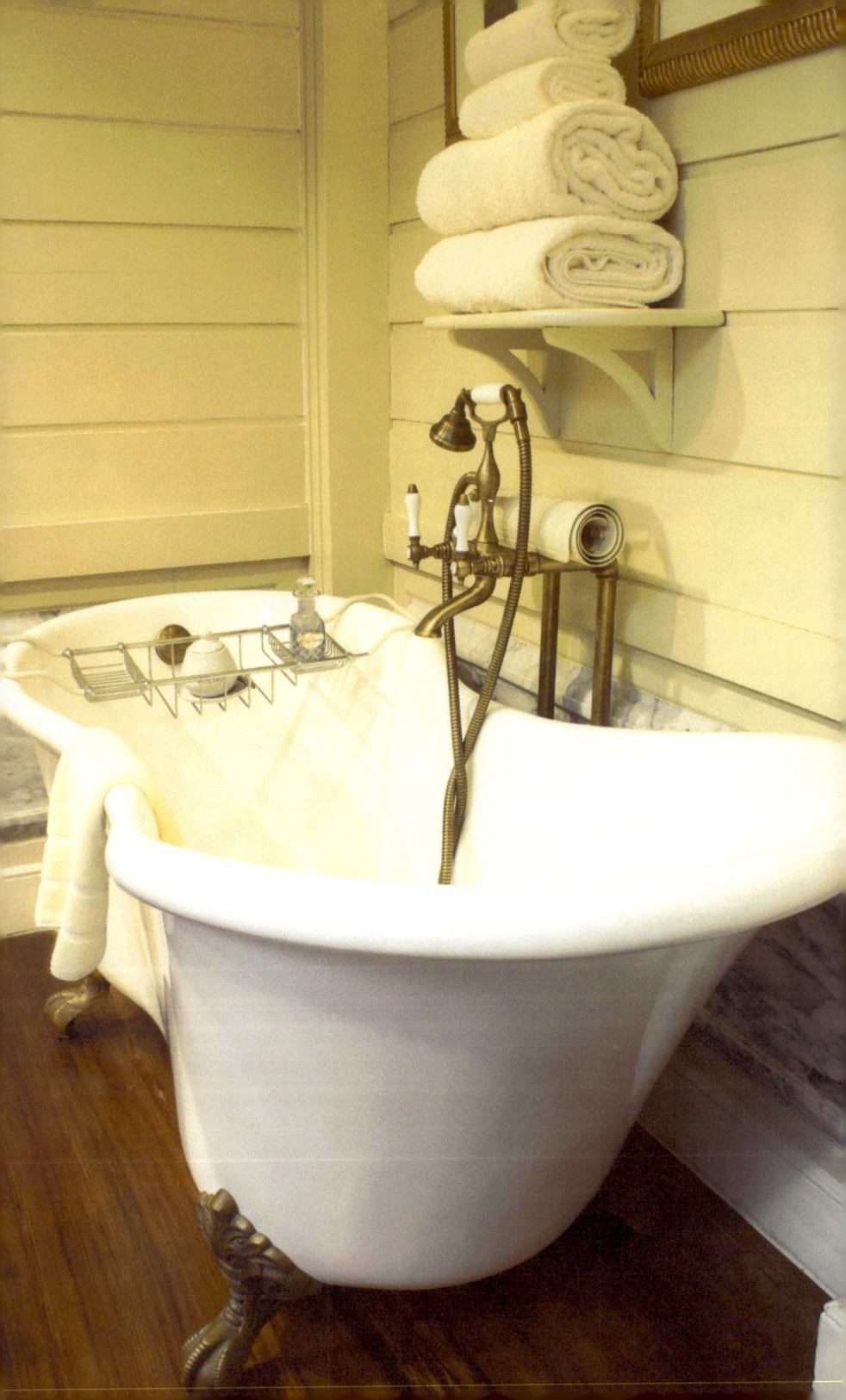

Sensitive skin needs special care. Your skin is very delicate and requires gentle cleaning practices and regular moisturizing. The skin is the body's largest organ and your first defense against disease. An important component of its defense mechanism is an waxy substance called sebum, which is secreted by the sebaceous gland. So many cleansers contain harsh chemicals like sodium lauryl sulfate and fragrances that break down this natural protective layer and further agitate the skin. It is best to avoid them and opt for natural cleansers instead.

bathing tips:

- Use a natural moisturizing body wash to nourish and gently cleanse your skin.

- Take short, warm showers and bath. Long hot baths and showers may feel good but are very drying

- Avoid harsh chemicals and irritating ingredients

- Apply a moisturizer immediately after showering to help to seal in moisture and keep your skin soft and supple.

- Use natural oils and butter such as shea butter, olive oil, coconut oil and jojoba oil to moisturize your skin. They contain fatty acids, anti-oxidants, vitamins, anti-inflammatories and nutrients that will improve your skin's health and make the symptoms of eczema more tolerable.

here is a **diy**
(Do-it-yourself)
recipe.

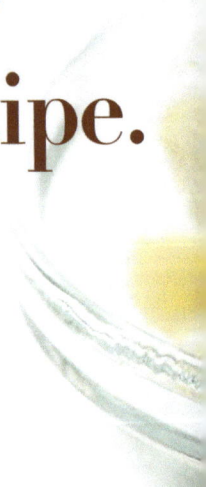

moisturizing
body butter

Ingredients -

- 1 cup of shea butter
- 1/4 cup of olive oil
- 1/4 cup of coconut oil

Directions - Warm the shea butter to make it easier to blend. Place all the ingredients into a mixing bowl and blend until completely incorporated and smooth. At this point you may add an essential oil or keep it unscented. Place the mixture in a jar and use daily to moisturize your skin.

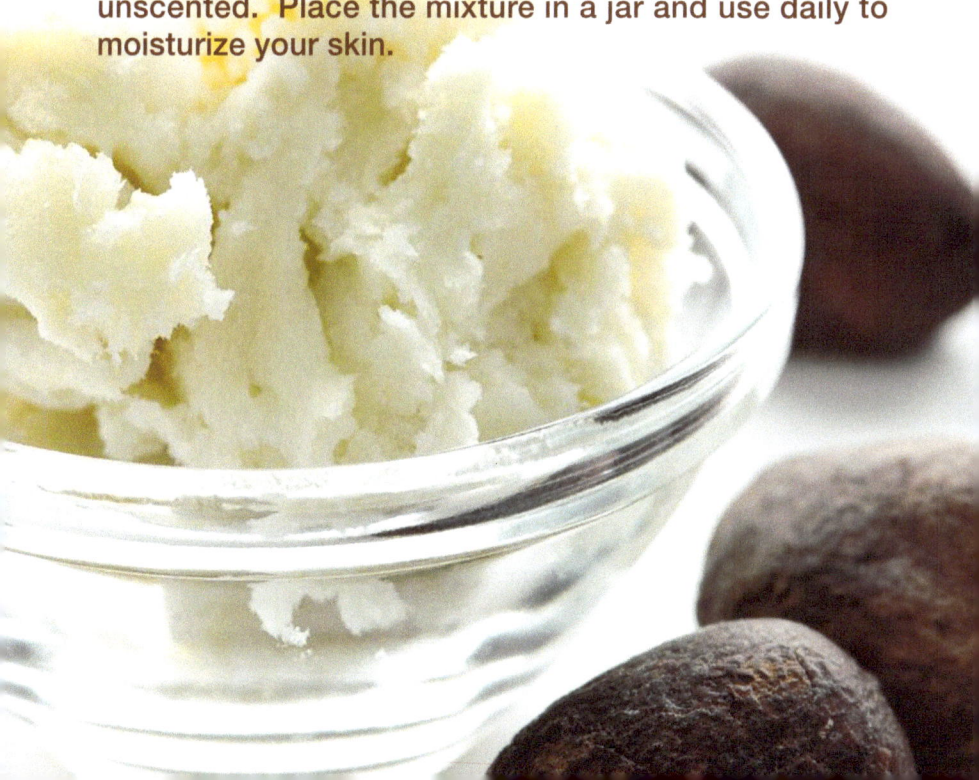

Nowadays you can find a variety of natural moisturizers and cleansers at most local health and beauty stores. Develop the habit of reading labels so you won't be mislead. A lot of companies are grasping at the natural health movement and use marketing and advertising ploys, like beautiful pictures of fruits and nuts on their packaging, to fool consumers into assuming its a natural product, while the product contains harsh chemicals and very little of the ingredients pictured.

read ingredients
labels
and avoid products that contain the following ingredients:

parabens
Common preservative found in most personal care items used to prevent the growth of bacteria and fungi. Some studies have suggested that this substance mimics hormonal activity in the body and can cause an increased risk of cancer.

phthalates
Found in fragrances, nail polish, hair spray, deodorants and perfumes. Phthalates has been shown to cause alterations in development and reduce testical size in males when subject is exposed to it in large doses.

DEA (cocamide DEA, Lauramide DEA, Linoleamide DEA and Oleamide DEA0-
Foaming agent found in most personal care items like shampoos, and body washes and can cause cancer

sodium lauryl sulfate
Foaming agent found in personal care items like shampoos, body washes and toothpaste which can cause skin and scalp irritation.

propylene glycol
Found in personal care items used to retain moisture; has been known to cause an eczema flare-up and trigger allergies.

bathing

17

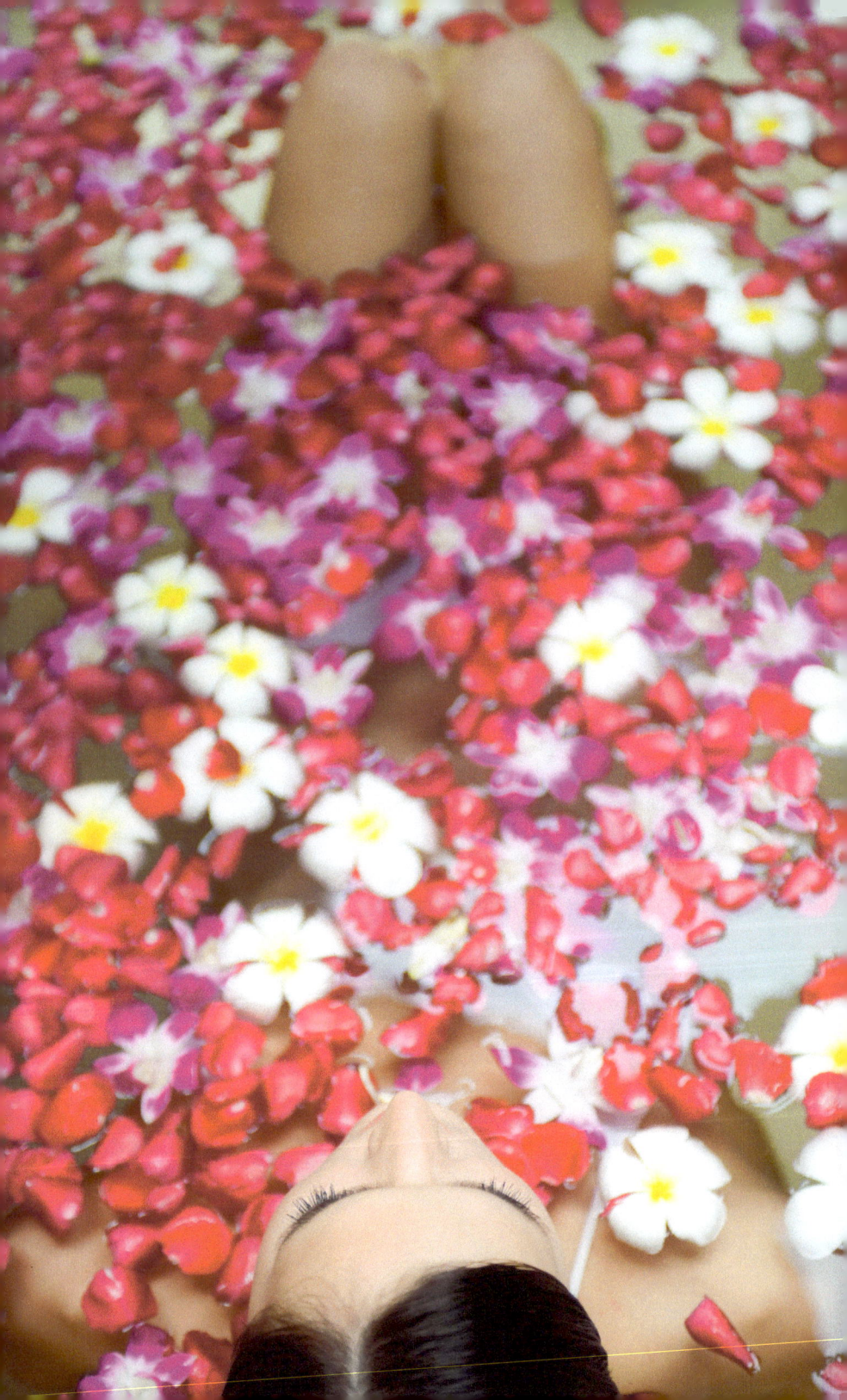

Soaking in a tub of warm water improves circulation, stimulates the lymphatic system, relaxes your muscles, and decrease stress.

Adding healing agents like herbs and essential oils to the bath water allows for it's distribution over a large area of the body, and is a great way to promote health and well being. Improving circulation also facilitates the transportation of oxygen and nutrients to the cells to support the healing process.

Excercise caution when bathing if you have a health issue that can be exacerbated by bathing. For example if you have hypertension sitting in a tub of hot water can dialate the blood vessels and cause a rapid drop in blood pressure, dizziness and fainting. Also, bathing in very hot water is contraindicated during pregnancy.

recipes for
soothing
bath
soaks.

18

be sure
the water is
warm
and not
hot.

Limit your soak time to ten to fifteen minutes.

If you have a health condition that may be exacerbated by bathing, please refrain.

These bath recipes are also a great way to take a moment out of your day to relax and enjoy some alone time. Don't forget to dim the lights, light some candles and put on some soothing music or grab a good book.

> Tip: You may use fresh or dried herbs. It's a good idea to place herbs in a mesh bag to prevent clogging the drain.

relaxing
bath soak

- 1/4 cup dried lavender buds
- 1/2 cup Dead sea salt
  (Do not use if you have open sores or cuts)
- 1 tbsp Honey
- 1/4 cup Coconut oil

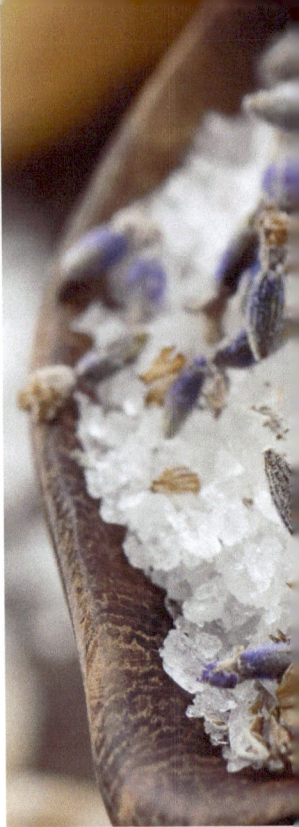

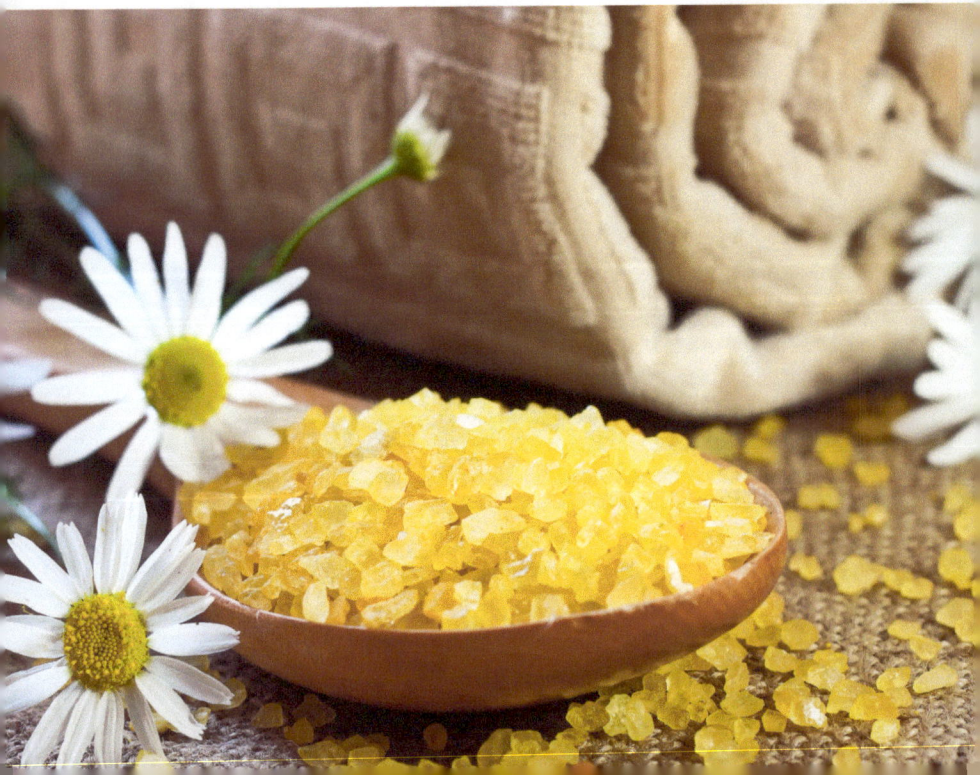

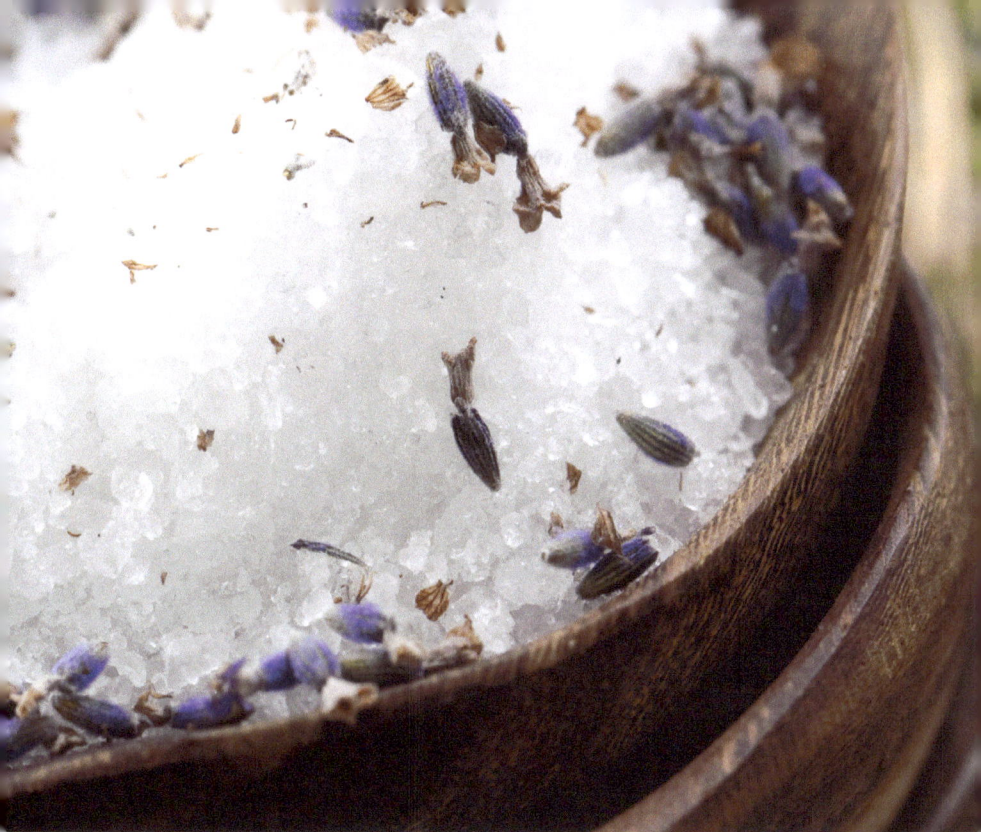

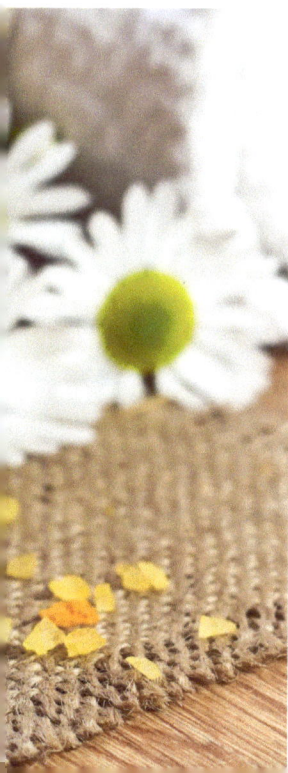

soothe
me now
bath soak

- 1/4 cup Chamomile
- 1/4 cup Oatmeal
- 1/4 cup Coconut oil

heal
me now
bath soak

- 1/2 cup Dead sea salt
  (Do not use if you have open sores or cuts)
- 1/4 cup Olive oil
- 1/4 cup Thyme
- 1/4 cup Sage

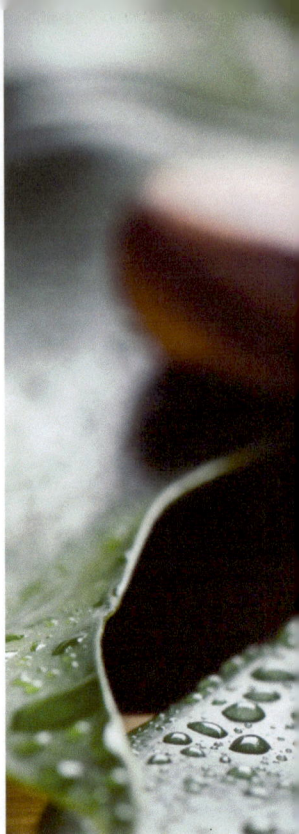

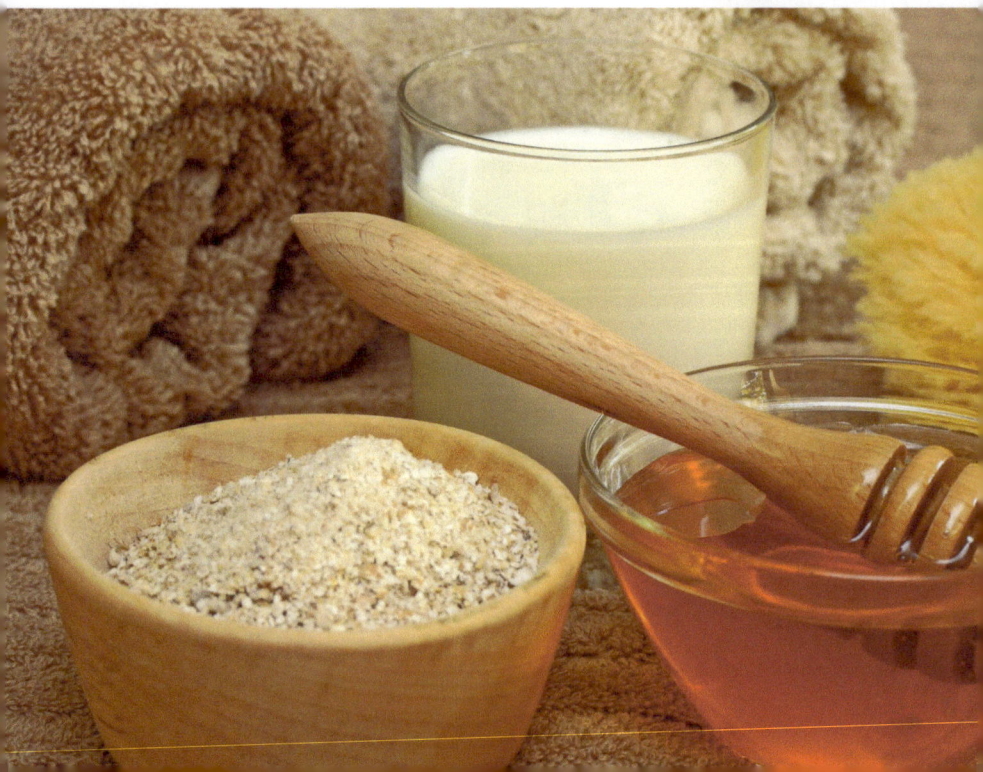

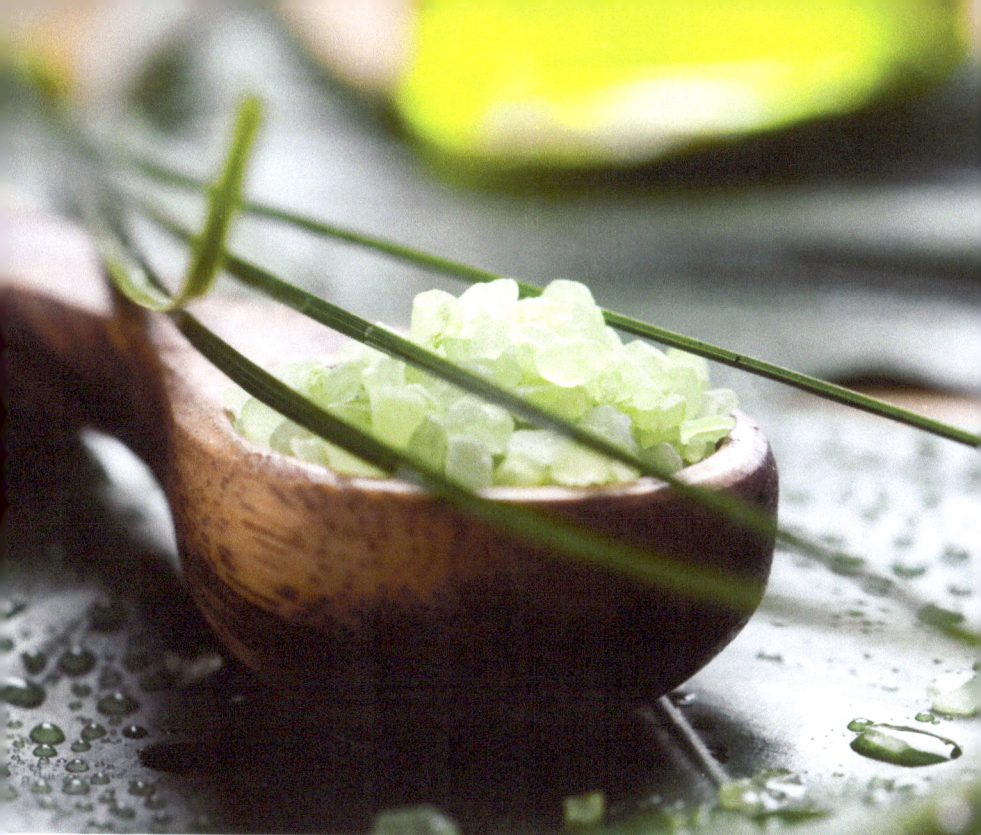

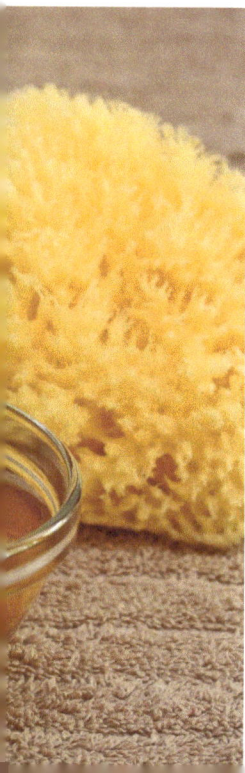

milk and honey
bath soak

- 1 cup powder milk
- 2 Tbsp honey
- 1 Tbsp vanilla extract
- 1 tsp cinnamon
- 1 cup almond oil

sore
no more
bath soak

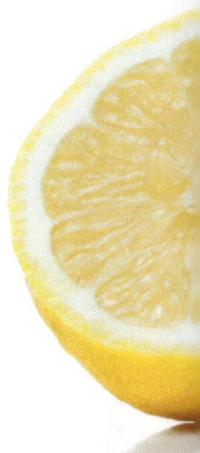

- 2 cups Epsom salt
  (skip if you have open sores or cuts)

- 2-3 drops peppermint oil

- 1 cup of olive oil

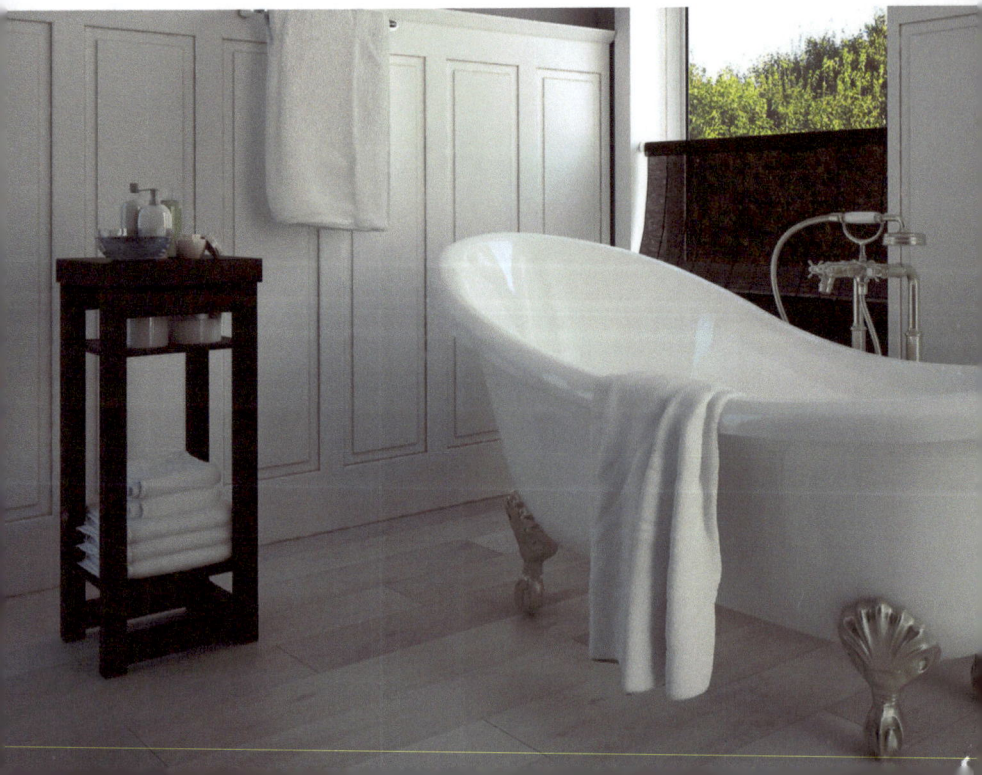

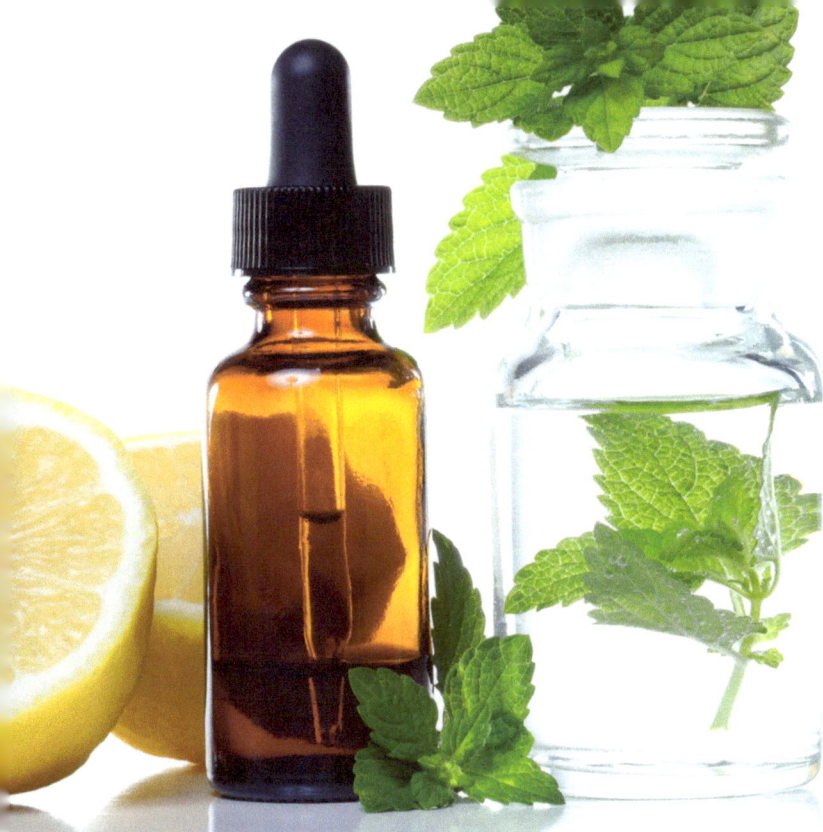

cider soak

My favorite for soothing itchy skin

Add two-three cups of apple cider vinegar to warm (not hot) bathwater and soak for fifteen to thirty minutes, following up with a cold rinse in the shower for one minute. Take these baths three to four times a week for best results.

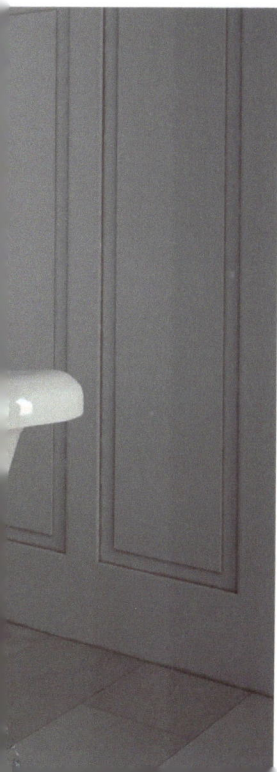

benefits of exfoliating

19

exfoliation

It takes approximately twenty-eight days for a skin cell to form and move from the dermis (lower level of the skin) to the epidermis (surface layer of the skin). The skin on the surface is actually dead, and naturally sloughs off as new skin cells surface. Exfoliating facilitates this process, keeps skin soft and supple, and evens skin tone.

There are several effective exfoliation techniques. One is dry brushing, a method in which you use a natural brush to remove dead skin cells, facilitate lymphatic drainage, improve circulation, and unclog pores.

Never exfoliate an active rash as it would be much like scratching the skin. This would worsen the rash and cause further damage

dry brushing

How often:

Dry brushing is something you can and should be doing daily. Even twice a day for healthy skin. Your skin should be dry, so the ideal time is in the shower before you turn on the water, so you don't get the brush wet.

Directions:

You should only brush towards the heart, making long sweeps. Avoid back and forth motions and scrubbing. Start at your feet, moving up the legs on both sides, then work from your arms toward your chest. On your stomach, direct the brush counter clockwise. And, don't brush too hard: skin should be stimulated and invigorated but not irritated or red.

Type of brush:

The bristles should be natural, not synthetic, and preferably vegetable derived. The bristles should be somewhat stiff, but not too hard. Look for a brush that has a long handle for hard-to-reach areas like your back.

Benefits:

In addition to sloughing away dry rough skin on knees, elbows, and ankles, dry brushing promotes firmer skin, stimulates new skin cell production and increases blood flow. It also helps the lymphatic system release toxins.

You'll notice a smoother complexion that glows. I love it because it's one of the easiest, cheapest, and most effective things you can do for promoting healthy skin.

scrubs

Another exfoliating technique is to use mildly abrasive natural ingredients like sugar or salt combined with natural oils and herbs to polish and nourish your skin. You can buy scrubs at local beauty stores or make them yourself at home.

How to use:

After taking a warm shower, apply scrub all over in a circular motion, making sure to pay attention to the rough spots, and rinse off thoroughly, pat dry to avoid removing skin nourishing oils. Be cautious when moving around the tub particularly when using scrubs with oils that can make surfaces slippery.

natural
exfoliates
you can make at home.

These natural exfoliating scrubs can easily be made in your kitchen to keep your skin soft and supple.

- Never exfoliate damaged or irritated skin, if a rash is present.

- Always apply to skin gently to avoid damage.

exfoliating scrubs

honey
cinnamon
scrub

- 1 cup Sugar
- 1 tsp Honey
- 2/3 cup Coconut oil
- 1 tsp ground cinnamon

citrus
polish

- 1 tbsp Grapefruit juice
- 1 cup Sugar
- 2/3 cup Sunflower oil

lemon
basil
scrub

- 1 cup Dead sea salt
- 2/3 cup Olive oil
- tbsp finely chopped Basil
- 2-3 drops Lemongrass

sweet
rosemary
lemon
scrub

- 2 tsp finely chopped rosemary
- 1 cup olive oil
- 1-2 drop essential oil of lemon
- 1 cup brown sugar
- 1 Tbsp honey

benefits of ingredients used in

diy

skin care recipes.

- ## lavender buds
  Stimulates new cell growth, aids in healing, relieves itching and has mild antiseptic properties

- ## dead sea salt
  High mineral content improves skin hydration and reduces inflammation *(avoid on broken skin).

- ## honey
  Natural humectant; improves skin hydration and aids in healing.

- ## coconut oil
  Excellent moisturizer, it easily penetrates skin leaving it soft and supple. Has antiseptic properties and promotes wound healing.

- ## chamomile
  Soothing and anti-inflammatory, are great at relieving eczema symptoms.

- ## oatmeal
  Soothes itching, gently cleanses and locks in moisture. It's anti-inflammatory and antioxidant properties are great for sensitive skin

- ## olive oil
  High in antioxidants, great for moisturizing dry skin

- ## thyme
  Powerful antiseptic, great skin toner

- ## sage
  Mild analgesic properties, stimulates cell growth, and increases circulation

- ## milk
  Contains lactic acid which greatly exfoliates and softens your skin.

- ## cinnamon
  Powerful anti-bacterial and antifungal agent, soothes achy muscles.

- ## almond oil
  Loaded with antioxidants and vitamin E and A, great for softening and relieving dry irritated skin.

- ## peppermint oil
  An antiseptic antibacterial cooling properties.
  (never use full strength on skin or on broken skin)

- ## grapefruit
  Evens skin tone, fights premature aging and tightens skin.

- ## sunflower oil
  An anti-aging agent high in vitamin E and omega 6 is a great anti-inflammatory.

- ## basil
  Antiseptic, that promotes wound healing.

- ## lemongrass
  Antibacterial, fungicidal, minimizes pores, improves circulation relieves pain and firms skin.

- ## rosemary
  Promotes cell regeneration and exfoliation, contains powerful disinfectant and antiseptic properties, lightens dark spots, reduces swelling and promotes healing.

- ## lemon
  Lightens dark spots, promotes healing and tones skin. Can also make skin sensitive to sunlight.

- ## shea butter
  Anti-inflammatory, powerful healing properties, promotes cell regeneration, reduces the appearances of scars, and has anti-aging properties.

20

internal remedies

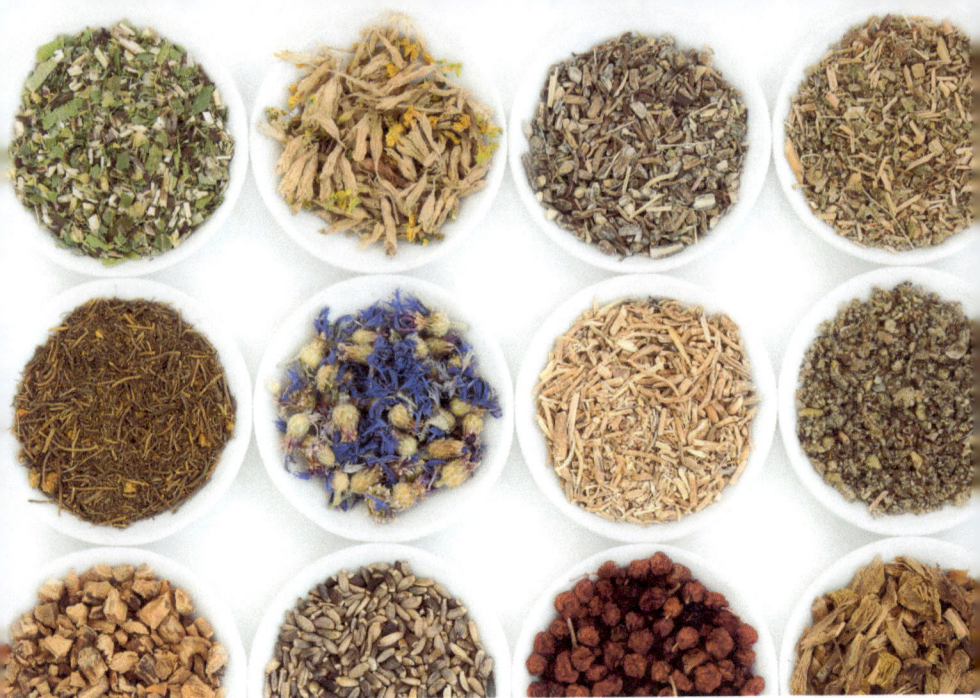

The following herbs support the body's natural ability to maintain health by stimulating and nourishing the body's cleansing organs; the lungs, kidneys, colon and skin. It's the job of these organs to remove harmful toxins and waste from the body.

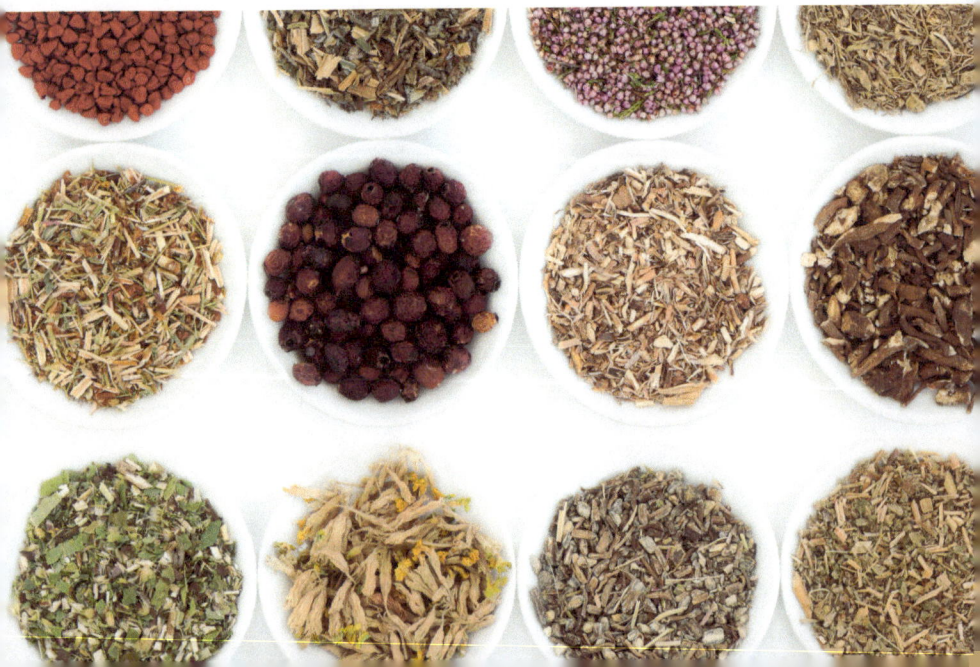

herbs
for cleansing

- ### dandelion root
  Supports liver function, helps regulate blood glucose levels and is an anti-inflammatory

- ### burdock root
  Blood purifier, diaphoretic (increase sweating), promotes kidney function to help clear the blood of harmful acids, anti-biotic and anti-fungal agent

- ### chickweed
  Is a cleansing herb that relieves blood toxicity, reduces inflammation and accelerates healing

- ### echinacea
  Binds to toxins in food and flushes them out, softens and dissolves harden masses of accumulated mucus
  * can be used topically to relieve eczema

- ### ginger root
  Stimulates circulation and enhances the cleansing mechanism of the skin, bowels and kidney

- ### golden seal root
  Antiseptic, anti-inflammatory and helps to promote healthy spleen and liver function
  * can be used topically to relieve eczema

- ### rhubarb root
  Clears bowel of accumulated fecal matter

- ### clove
  Anti-inflammatory, antiseptic, improves respiratory health and aids in digestion
  * can be used topically to relieve eczema

- ### valerian
  Eases nervous tension, insomnia and stress

  * Use caution when taking anything while pregnant
  ** Consult your physician

how to make

herbal
tea

Herbal tea can be made using fresh or dry herbs. Steep fresh herbs for no more than 3 minutes and dried herbs for 4-6 minutes. Simply bring water to a boil, then pour it over the herbs, cover and let it sit. Add lemon and/or honey for taste and the added benefit of the high vitamin C content of lemons and the added benefits. Lemons are high in vitamin C and honey has anti-septic properties.

Some tea can also be used topically on the skin to relieve inflamed skin conditions. When using topically, allow tea to cool. I like to place a cup of tea made with golden seal in the refrigerator to get it nice and cold. Then I use a cotton ball to apply it to my skin. This is great for relieving itchy skin and reducing inflammation as well as preventing infection.

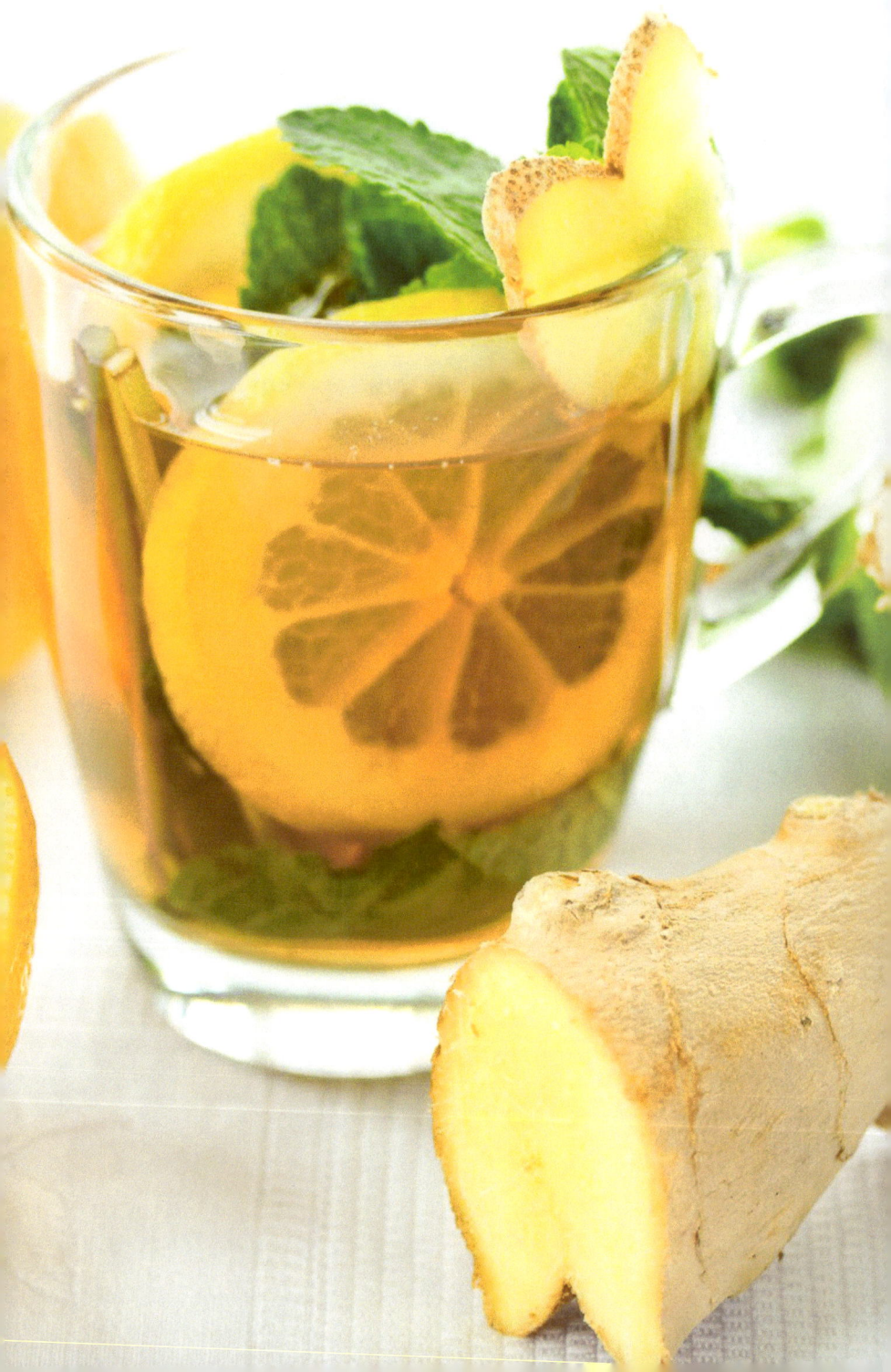

tonics

an agent which has properties that restores balance

apple cider vinegar tonic

Apple cider vinegar (ACV) is a powerful cleansing and healing elixir. It's alkalinity helps to maintain the normal ph of the blood. It supports the body's natural detoxification process by stimulating the liver and the lymphatic system. It also assist in the removal of accumulated mucous throughout the body.

* 1-2 Tbsp of apple cider vinegar in one 8oz glass of water 1-2 times a day.
** Optional - Add honey for taste

lemon tonic

Lemon juice molecular structure is similar to the body's digestive juices. It aids in digestion, improves waste elimination and enhances immunity. Another added plus is that it's an alkalizing properties restore Blood ph balance.

* Squeeze fresh lemon juice into a glass of warm water.

21
in conclusion

Eczema is so complicated because of it's non-specific nature. The triggers and severity varies greatly from one person to the next. Consequently, what provides one person with relief may have no effect on you.

Be patient and remember that the body has an amazing, innate ability to heal itself. When you get a cut, there is no conscious effort on your part to form a scab, it just happens. Much like you don't have to remember to breathe or to have your heart beat. When your mind, body and spirit are in harmony you have the ability to naturally heal yourself.

Remember this as you begin to

nurture yourself
naturally

resources

Dietary Intervention in eczema
Paediatrics and Child Health, Volume 21, Issue 9, September 2011,
Pages 406-410\
Jackelina Pando Kelly, Jonathan Hourihan

Atopic Dermatitis: Update and Proposed Management Algorithm
Actas Dermo-Sifiliográficas (English Edition), Volume 104, Issue 1,
January–February 2013, Pages 4-16
G. Garnacho-Saucedo, R. Salido-Vallejo, J.C. Moreno-Giménez

Management of Difficult-to-Treat Atopic Dermatitis
Original Research Article
The Journal of Allergy and Clinical Immunology: In Practice, Volume 1,
Issue 2, March 2013, Pages 142-151
Peter D. Arkwright, Cassim Motala, Hamsa Subramanian, Jonathan
Spergel, Lynda C. Schneider, Andreas Wollenberg, Atopic Dermatitis
Working Group of the Allergic Skin Diseases Committee of the AAAAI

Prospective observational study of 42 patients with atopic dermatitis
treated with homeopathic medicines
Original Research Article
Homeopathy, Volume 101, Issue 1, January 2012, Pages 21-27
José Enrique Eizayaga, Juan Ignacio Eizayaga

The problem of atopic eczema: aetiological clues from the
environment and lifestyles Original Research Article
Social Science & Medicine, Volume 46, Issue 6, 1 March 1998,
Pages 729-741
N.J. McNally, D.R. Phillips, H.C. William

Epidemiology.
2012 May;23(3):4012-14. doi: 10.1097/EDE.0b013e31824d5da2.

Probiotics supplementation during pregnancy or infancy for the
prevention of atopic dermatitis: a meta-analysis.

Pelucchi C1, Chatenoud L, Turati F, Galeone C, Moja L, Bach JF, La
Vecchia C.

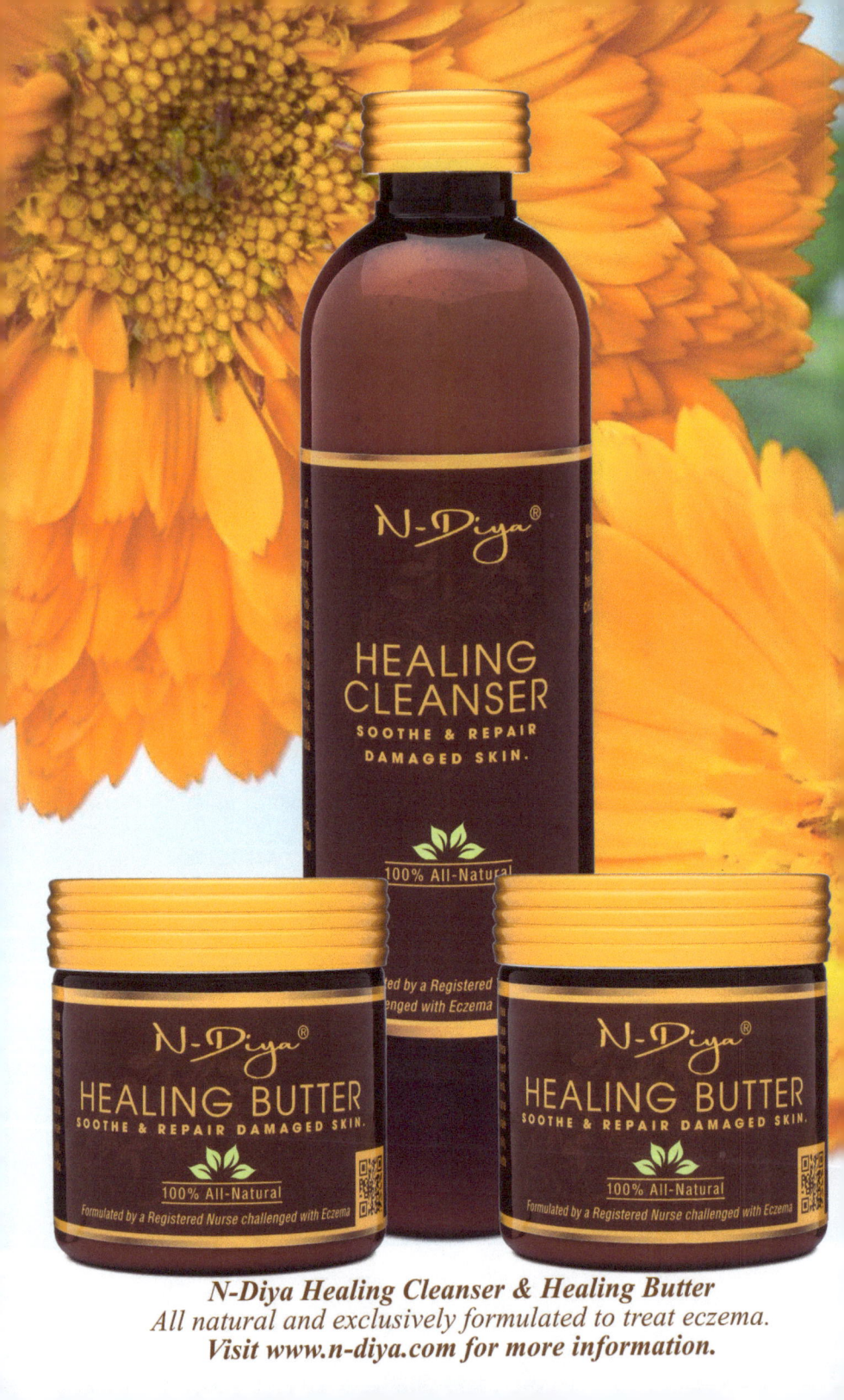

N-Diya Healing Cleanser & Healing Butter
All natural and exclusively formulated to treat eczema.
Visit www.n-diya.com for more information.